Praise for Barbara Savin

"Science tells us that energy is real. It can't be created, and it can't be destroyed, but it can be harnessed. Barbara has a very blessed way of moving energy. She is a servant of goodwill and promoting light."
—PHARRELL WILLIAMS

"We all have the power and ability to heal ourselves. Through Barbara, I have discovered what energy work is and can do—within us and surrounding us. Learning how to engage and shift that energy has allowed me to embrace a deeper sense of inner calm, balance, and peace in my life."
—CHRISTINA AGUILERA

"Everything a reader needs to know to embrace the practice of gentle energy healing."
—PUBLISHERS WEEKLY

"A fantastic book for anyone curious about energy healing. This is the book I was looking for thirty years ago when I began my journey as a psychic medium and healer. Barbara Savin does a beautiful job of sharing, teaching, and validating experiences that are otherwise unexplainable to many people stepping into this new realm of awareness. Years of experience and insight have given Barbara an amazing understanding of something so subtle yet powerful: our ability to heal ourselves. This is the secret that is ready to be unleashed, and thanks to Barbara, the information is now available to anyone willing to read it."
—SUNNY DAWN JOHNSTON, author of *Invoking the Archangels* and *The Love Never Ends: Messages from the Other Side*

"I have always been a spiritual person, so when my good friend and counselor suggested I see an energy healer, I was intrigued. The universe in its infinite wisdom led me to Barbara. The moment we met, I felt her beautiful, caring spirit and knew we would achieve spiritual health and growth together. Barbara helped me focus my energy in a positive, healing way. This gave me the clarity and strength needed to work on the issues at hand. I felt blessed in love and light, which, in turn, allowed me to bless those who were struggling. I've worked with Barbara for over two years. I've sent countless friends to her when they needed healing and guidance. They have all felt what I experienced. Barbara is a pure and gentle soul, a loving and gifted teacher. Beauty and light pour out of her, and I'm thrilled that she will be able to share her gifts with others through this book."

—PAT BENATAR, four-time Grammy winner and author of *Between a Heart and a Rock Place*

"Barbara Savin is one of the finest energy healers I have ever had the pleasure of working with. Not only is she an inspired and magnificent teacher, but Barbara is also a remarkable healer. Her approach is gentle and loving, yielding incredibly powerful results. In her new book, Barbara graciously shares her remarkable gifts with all her readers in a fresh, unique, and insightful style. Truly, she is a rare and precious woman, with the Grace of God flowing through her heart and soul."

—HEATHER MCCLOSKEY BECK, inspirational speaker and author of *Take the Leap*

"Barbara is a true healer. She tuned right in to my needs in a gentle and compassionate way. After meeting with her, my body, mind, and spirit felt lighter and clearer. I have recommended many people to her, and all have felt as I do about her amazing talents."

—SUE GLASSCOCK, owner, The Ranch at Live Oak Malibu

"Barbara Savin is an extraordinary energy healer. I have referred friends, family, and patients to her for years, and I have always been amazed at the results. This book will benefit everyone who reads it. I give her and her book the highest recommendation."
                —SHARON NORLING, MD, MBA, author of *Your Doctor Is Wrong*

"I have had the pleasure of working with Barbara for nearly ten years and have found her care of patients to be outstanding. She has a remarkable ability to bond with her patients through her empathy and charm. Her level of expertise and ability with energy healing and clinical hypnotherapy is unmatched and has helped so many patients through the years. I'm sure this book will be a wonderful tool for those interested in energy healing in the years to come.
                —JONATHAN R. COLE, MD, managing partner, California Health
                & Longevity Institute

"Barbara Savin is an inspiring teacher, healer, and author. Her energy healing method works. She inspires many people to heal themselves and others. This book is a true gift to people who want to learn more about the art of healing. Barbara is gifted with the ability to teach this material; her book is easy to read, and her methods are easy to learn. Highly recommended!"
                —MARILYN GORDON, life transformation teacher and author of
                Healing Is Remembering

"Barbara Savin is the most intuitive, kindhearted, and empowering person I know. Her energy healing work has changed my life. Thanks to her, I feel more connected than I ever have to myself and more capable of tapping into my personal connection to the universe. She has given me a renewed sense of inner strength that has taken me to new levels in my personal life and in my career."
                —LINDSAY RUSH, songwriter and music executive

Gentle Energy Touch

The Beginner's Guide to Hands-On Healing

Barbara E. Savin, C.ht.

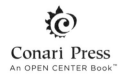

Conari Press
An OPEN CENTER Book™

This edition first published in 2016 by Conari Press, an imprint of
Red Wheel/Weiser, LLC
With offices at:
65 Parker Street, Suite 7
Newburyport, MA 01950
www.redwheelweiser.com

ISBN: 978-1-57324-679-8

Library of Congress Cataloging-in-Publication Data

Names: Savin, Barbara E., 1948-
Title: Gentle energy touch : the beginner's guide to hands-on healing /
  Barbara E. Savin, C. Ht.
Description: Newburyport, MA : Conari Press, an imprint of Red Wheel/Weiser,
  LLC, 2016.
Identifiers: LCCN 2015046802 | ISBN 9781573246798 (6 x 9 tp : alk. paper)
Subjects: LCSH: Energy medicine. | Touch—Therapeutic use. | Mind and body
  therapies. | Massage.
Classification: LCC RZ421 .S275 2016 | DDC 615.8/52—dc23
LC record available at http://lccn.loc.gov/2015046802

Cover design by Jim Warner
Cover photograph © Nikki Zalewski
Interior by Maureen Forys, Happenstance Type-O-Rama
Typeset in Adobe Garamond Pro

The positions found in chapters 7–9 were created and photographed by Barbara E. Savin and demonstrated by Denise Capri, Jenna Capri, Joan Mazzeo-Little, and Barbara E. Savin. The video links at the end of the book were created by Barbara E. Savin, filmed by Jennifer King, and demonstrated with Hayley Bianchi. Thank you to the Four Seasons Hotel located at Two Dole Drive, Westlake Village, California, for allowing us to film in their massage room. Grateful acknowledgment is made to Denise, Jenna, Joan, Jennifer, and Hayley for permission to use these photographs and video link in this book.

The MP3 links at the back of the book—Relax, Restore, Rebalance, Building Self-Confidence, and Empower Your Potential—were recorded and written by Barbara E. Savin, with music by Dr. Christopher Lloyd Clarke, BSc, MscD, meditation music composer and founder of RoyaltyFreeMeditationMusic.com.

Printed in Canada
MAR

10 9 8 7 6 5 4 3 2 1

To my family, friends, and spiritual teachers,
and those seeking truth and love.

I thank everyone who has touched my soul
and helped to show me the way.

May God bless you and always protect you.

Unconditionally loving is what life is all about.

Trusting the love of God has been reborn in me.

Thank you, God. I Love You.

CONTENTS

穏
気
触

INTRODUCTION

How I Discovered the Healing Power of Gentle Energy Touch

Energy healing is a gift I knew about from an early age, yet only fully explored when my body needed healing physically, emotionally, and spiritually. I grew up in Coney Island in Brooklyn, NY and my Grandma Jenny would always do healings on my sister and me.

We would sit quietly in a chair, and Grandma would ask for God's healing energy for us. She would begin at the top of our heads and in a slow sweeping motion, clear our energy and send it to either God or Mother Earth with love. Then she would lay her hands on our shoulders asking God to keep us healthy and safe. We would always feel heat and/or tingling coming from her hands, and my sister and I thought Grandma had magical powers. There were occasions when she would burn cloves and clear us with the smoke instead of using her healing hands. I remember Grandma always saying to us: "Think positive and trust in God's healing and always protect your energy. Always put God's healing light around you to protect you from negativity. Never allow anyone's words to bring you down . . . allow those words to fall to the ground." We were never sick and would always say, "Grandma, please stop doing healing so we can get sick and stay home from school!" But she never listened. She just continued to heal and clear us.

It is May 1966, just days away from my graduation from Lafayette High School in Brooklyn. I have been looking forward to this day for years. I am graduating with honors and receiving the Mayor's Award. I am picturing my Grandma Jenny sitting in the audience. I can imagine the pride on her face as I stand up when my name is called to receive this award. I am so excited; I plan to get a job right after graduation and buy her anything she wants. I love my grandma with all my heart. And then I find out the worst news of my young life. At two o'clock in the morning, our family receives a phone call telling us that Grandma Jenny has died.

How could this be? She was only sixty-four. She was supposed to be alive to celebrate my most important day, and now she was gone. The news broke my heart; I felt so angry with God. Why did he take this woman who loved me so much? Why did he take her before my important day? My time with her was just beginning. I felt that this was so unfair, and the more I wept for her, the more I lost my faith and trust in God.

About two weeks later, graduation now behind me, I was alone at home when I heard a voice calling out to me. I thought this must be my imagination; only Grandma called me "Babasita," and that's what I was hearing. I got up from the chair and began walking to the foyer. There, I saw a white cloud and heard again, softly but clearly, "Babasita."

I said, "Grandma, Grandma, is that you?"

And she replied, "Yes, Babasita, everything is okay. Don't be so angry, Babasita." The closer I got to the cloud, the more clearly I could see her.

I became frightened and ran to the phone to call my mother, who was away visiting her brother. Over the phone, my mom told me I was hearing Grandma's voice because I missed her so much. I was supposed to believe that my grief had created this entire episode. My mom and I never spoke about this again—nor any other "unnatural" experiences I had, including my ability to do healings just like my grandma.

Angry about my grandma's death, I decided I would no longer do healings and stopped helping two of my close friends who had never made fun of my ability. I simply said to them: "I am sorry, but I do not believe in God's healing anymore." Also, when I saw spirits or heard a voiceless voice, I would say, "You are not real; go away and stop speaking to me. Leave me alone." This, I thought, was my way of punishing God. However, as the years went on, my body began to break down. I was constantly sick, always stressed, working at a job I disliked plus raising two children. One day, my niece Stefanie happened to see a flyer mentioning a Reiki healing circle. Neither of us knew what Reiki was, but since we were both in poor shape physically and emotionally, we decided to go to the healing circle in Staten Island.

The atmosphere there was wonderful. Everyone sang songs of love, and it was so calm and peaceful. The practitioners did Reiki work on us, and the feeling was like nothing I had experienced except with my grandma and her healings. I sat and cried and instantly knew that I had to take this up again.

From that moment on, I knew that energy healing was what I needed to do; it felt so natural to me. For the first time, I understood the need to help myself heal from within. I remained focused and did self-healings at least twice a day for a month. I could feel changes, even though my body pain had gotten worse. I recognized I hated and loved myself at the same time. I was going through a lot spiritually, and I realized I hadn't forgiven my grandma as thoroughly as I thought I had. I knew I still needed to work on that part of myself. Most importantly, I had to begin loving myself for who I am at my core: a healer.

And while I also knew in my heart that I was a healer, I found it difficult to express that to others. Remember that this was 1960s

New York. I recalled how my grandma would always say, "Shush, don't tell anyone about my healings because they'll put us away in a crazy hospital." I knew I had intuitive abilities and was able to feel people's energies, and I often saw or sensed spirits, but I was so afraid that people would think I was crazy if I talked about it. Meanwhile, my body was crying out for healing and for me to allow my passion and purpose to come forward. This was not an easy task, and I will say that it did not happen overnight. It took time and patience.

First Healing Miracle . . .

Giving myself healing treatments made me realize that the pain I was experiencing was not only physical but also rooted in emotional and spiritual challenges. Then a miracle happened.

At the time, I was experiencing black particles floating in front of my eyes, making it hard to see. I was frightened and very stressed. One morning, while looking in the mirror and speaking to myself, I asked God for assistance. I asked God to help me understand what was happening and to please make the black particles go away.

Suddenly I heard a voice within me say, "All you need to do is ask," and immediately the black particles disappeared. In that very moment, I realized God does listen and speak to us, but we often choose not to hear. God sees and understands us, but we often choose not to see nor understand ourselves. God loves us unconditionally, but we often choose to love with conditions. Once I truly began believing in God again, more miracles happened. My body became pain free and my chronic fatigue a thing of the past. No more headaches, no more pain, and I actually lost some weight. I felt human again. I was able to love and be happy with myself.

That was when I committed to deepening my knowledge of healing. I studied pranic healing and hypnotherapy, became a meditation instructor, and learned Reiki and Healing Touch. When I would give or receive a healing, I now experienced a sense of complete peacefulness. My inner being felt centered and balanced, filled with God's white light. I felt a oneness with everything in existence—people, birds, bugs, animals, grass, trees, air, ocean, sky, and the universe. I felt love in my heart for all creation—including myself. I was filled with the desire to share that feeling with others and knew that if I touched just one person with the loving energy of God, I would have made a difference in the world.

That was in 1999. Then two years later, on September 11, 2001, my healing abilities were put to the test. I remember watching the television news reports in horror, witnessing the second plane hit the World Trade Center and then the collapse of both buildings. I started shaking uncontrollably, overcome with anxiety and panic as I feared the worst. Then I heard a voice coming from within myself, telling me, "Calm yourself; do your healing. Trust that everything will be fine."

You see, my son and my husband worked across the street from the Twin Towers and always had breakfast inside the Twin Towers every morning at that time. Through all the stress and fear, I asked God for his healing energy and gently put my hands on my heart to calm myself. I knew the situation was completely out of my control, and I began to pray not just for my two but for everyone.

After hours of not knowing their fate, I got a call from my husband and son; they were all right—very sad and shaken but alive. I was so grateful to the universe that I dropped all my fear of coming out as a healer. I started volunteering at various health centers and hospitals, helping those with HIV, AIDS, and cancer.

I volunteered to do hospice care. And I started showing up to help out at the tent the Salvation Army put up on Staten Island for all the workers involved in the 9/11 recovery and rescue.

I was asked to do a meditation for over 350 girls at St. Peter's Catholic High School so they could feel safe after 9/11. I knew in my heart that I needed to help people to help themselves to heal, and, in turn, the world would be a better place in which to live.

A few years into this new chapter of my life, we moved to California to be with our grandchildren. Shortly thereafter, nearly ten years ago now, I was hired to be the energy healing specialist and clinical hypnotherapist at the then brand-new California Health & Longevity Institute in The Four Seasons Hotel in Westlake Village. I was also hired to work with renowned Sharon Norling, MD, author of *Your Doctor Is Wrong,* at the Mind, Body, and Spirit Center in Westlake Village, helping her clients. Once *I* began to truly believe, my life changed.

My grandma may not have been there for my graduation, but I know she sees me now. She comes to me, and I am able to feel her presence and hear her. I express my deep love for her and tell her how much I miss her and thank her for showing me how to heal. I now realize that God needed her to help others and that it was important for her to be on the other side. I finally have forgiven myself, my Grandma Jenny, and God. I am free to be me.

At this point, I have been practicing energy healing for about sixteen years and have been blessed to work with thousands of clients suffering from any kind of physical, emotional, or spiritual issue imaginable. I have helped many people release the root cause of their challenges. Through my energy healing and hypnosis/meditation work, I have seen people regain a sense of calm and balance, physically and emotionally. I have seen people helped with their heart disease and cancer, their skin problems, cuts, bruises, back pain, depression, anxiety, and everything else. I have seen how energy work complements all medical modalities, accelerates treatment, and speeds healing.

It is wonderful, miraculous work, and I am blessed to be able to do it. I have also done a lot of healing work with dogs, our divine companions. More on that in my next book . . .

Gentle Energy Touch

I have come to call what I do Gentle Energy Touch, and that's what I'm going to teach you in this book. Anyone can do it. It becomes more and more powerful with practice, of course, so don't get discouraged if you don't see dramatic results quickly. Keep at it, and the healing will come.

I don't know where my grandma learned to heal—possibly from her own mother who was born in Istanbul. But there's certainly nothing new about hands-on healing. It is an ancient method of revitalizing the energy fields of your own (or someone else's) body. I'm going to start at the beginning and teach you each of the basic techniques in turn. We'll create a solid foundation and then build from there. We'll start with things you can do for your own healing, and then I will show you how to use these techniques on family and friends. If you are already an energy practitioner, I think you will find plenty of information here that will be useful as well.

You will learn hands-on techniques to target specific areas of the body that need attention. Most important, you will learn how to apply Gentle Energy Touch with the intention of asking for Divine/Universal Energy, the force that revitalizes our own life force and helps us heal.

Perhaps you've gotten good results from alternative therapies such as meditation, yoga, exercise, improved diet, acupuncture and acupressure, and/or reflexology and massage. There are also other touch therapies or energy healing techniques, such as Reiki, Healing Touch, etc. All of these approaches work because they unblock life force energy. There are many extraordinary healers in the world who have dedicated their lives to understanding how we become ill and helping us stay well, but the truth is, anyone with the desire to maintain and stay healthy can easily learn to tap into this energy. No license is required—just practice. You can improve your own health once you understand how.

We'll start by looking at the seven major chakras that are so critical to maintaining our health. Our chakras work like valves that allow life force energy to flow in and out of us and circulate throughout the physical, mental, emotional, and spiritual parts of our being, helping balance our body's systems. Even conventional Western medicine is beginning to embrace the fact that we are not simply physical parts and functions and that there are energy fields (auras) that surround the body and energy centers (chakras) within the body, all of which can become imbalanced, whether by stress or trauma or injury or simply by inattention. Our goal is to restore balance to the chakras and auras.

When our auras and chakras are weakened or blocked, we are more likely to get sick. When they are strong and free-flowing, it is easier to maintain our health and well-being. Learning how to cleanse and balance the chakras will help you understand why you may have an illness, offer a way to resolve the "issues in your tissues," and heal. This cleansing opens the door to creating a healthier body, mind, and spirit. What this is all about, really, is taking responsibility for your own healing. And if your life's lesson *is* the illness, learning about the chakras will help you understand why you are going through your particular challenges.

Think about it: Why is it that two people can be exposed to the same toxic environment and one becomes ill while the other does not? Why is it that of all those who smoke, only some get emphysema or lung cancer and others stay healthy? Why is it that some people develop diabetes at an early age and others eat sugar all day long yet do not have a problem until later in life? Why do some people get depressed and others always seem to have a positive outlook? The answers to these questions are in this book. Not only will you understand *why* things are the way they are, you will discover that you have the power to change them—to help heal your own body, take steps to prevent illness, and be in better control of your own wellness.

Imagine being able to utilize the power of your mind for healing just by asking. Gentle Energy Touch uses intention alone to begin the healing process and activates when your hands are placed on your body. You will learn that the energy that seems so mysterious and obscure is quite simple and readily available to you just for the asking. It is with you all of the time for the rest of your life. Gentle Energy Touch can be learned by any-one who is open and willing to allow this healing energy to flow through their body. It amazes me how energy healing truly works on all levels—physical, mental, emotional, and spiritual—truly supporting our inner growth and spiritual development. You will learn the beginning techniques that will help you build a strong foundation so there is no doubt in your mind that you can help yourself and others to heal.

By learning and giving yourself Gentle Energy Touch treatments on a regular basis, you will notice that your once-frazzled energy is now centered, grounded, and balanced. You will notice that your mind is more at peace and your everyday stress-ors are easier to deal with. Gentle Energy Touch will help you enjoy healthier relationships with others and allow you to heal emotional and mental wounds that no longer serve your purpose. Learning this technique will reduce your stress, giving you the ability to see things more clearly and make better decisions that will foster your fulfillment and happiness. These are just some of the benefits of Gentle Energy Touch that will be discussed in this book. I would like to mention here that you are in the right place, right now, and this is the time for you to learn this ancient technique now being offered in medical institutes, hospitals, wellness centers, spas, and hotels—because it works!

The key to healing lies in enhancing your life force energy so your immune system will get stronger and you will feel more energized, have improved sleep, and so much more. You must realize that you must do the work for yourself. In order to feel like you have never felt before, you have to do something that you have never done before: change. This is about all aspects of yourself on all levels. Give it a go if you want to be healthy, happy, successful, and fulfill your life's purpose and passion.

I want to mention here that energy healing can save lives. It saved mine many years ago when I was diagnosed with crippling arthritis, chronic fatigue, and migraines. When you choose to let go of your challenges and learn to forgive and accept, energy healing can save your life, too, whether you need physical, mental, emotional, or spiritual healing. From my own experience, I can say there are no limits to what energy healing can accomplish, provided it is in line with the soul's life plan. If your journey is the illness, energy healing will enable you to understand why this is happening. Through my experiences with thousands of clients, I have seen energy healing face some of the darkest sources of emotional and physical pain a human body can withstand and win, lifting the weight of that pain, providing relief for the patients, helping them become the best versions of themselves, and enabling them to fulfill their true life purpose. That is why I have devoted my life to teaching and to writing this book.

Who Can Benefit from Gentle Energy Touch?

Gentle Energy Touch is good for everyone! Its goal is to discover the limitation causing a blockage, recognize its pattern and where it comes from, and then let it go. Letting go allows the body, mind, and spirit to heal. Once you understand and release your limitations, the growth and healing process is set in motion. Life commences in a way you have never experienced before. Everyone in need of healing in any form will truly benefit from this therapeutic modality.

Gentle Energy Touch is particularly useful for doctors, nurses, psychologists, therapists, and all care providers who wish to bring touch and deeper caring into their healing practices.

Patients in intensive care units or in any hospital environment can benefit greatly from Gentle Energy Touch, especially when human contact is important. Patients can feel comforted and attended by a compassionate person.

Babies, small children, and even animals are especially receptive to this energy since they have not developed defensive tendencies. They are automatically more open to loving energy.

The elderly and sick can benefit greatly from Gentle Energy Touch on many levels. Our society works in such a way that many of our older generation find themselves on their own, whether through the breakup of their family structure, the death of a partner, having no children to assist them, or other reasons. Many live alone, far from relatives, in elderly housing or retirement communities. As a result of being alone much of the time, they can suffer from feelings of depression, disorientation, loneliness, and lack of self-worth.

When their enjoyment of life diminishes, they tend to get sick frequently, potentially becoming bedridden. Replenishing life force energy with Gentle Energy Touch can help these individuals heal emotionally, mentally, physically, and spiritually, giving them a greater sense of peace and helping them to better cope on their own.

Gentle Energy Touch can provide support and comfort, and make the transition easier for a person who is dying. You can hold the dying person's hand and treat him/her with Gentle Energy Touch. The protection, acceptance, and understanding of the process provide a calmness that allows individuals to transition peacefully. I know this because I assisted not only in my mom's passing but also helped many others pass on, including my best friend Joan. My mom allowed me to do healing on her, knowing she would feel safe, protected, and at peace during her transititon.

It is important for you to realize that you are already a healer. Our ancestors were able to heal themselves and others without any special training because back then, they were more regularly in touch with their higher self and unified field. However, because of so much negativity around us from the media, Internet, wars, etc., we need to get back to understanding our own abilities to heal. It is time to rid our bodies of congestion from the stuck energy that causes us to be physically ill. Energy depletion needs to be counteracted. I will show you how to help yourself renew, refresh, and rebalance your energy field and your life!

As I see it,

Healing is a choice. Only you can make the decision to move toward optimum health.

Healing is a way of life. Only you can develop the ways to be healthy and happy.

Healing is channeling. Only you can embrace the flow of positive energy through you for a healthier body.

Healing is knowledge. Knowing the integration of your body, mind, and spirit will have a positive impact on your state of health.

Healing is accepting. Only you can accept responsibility and take charge of your own life.

Healing is love. The key is to love and accept yourself—your whole self.

Life presents a continuous flow of experiences and challenges that trigger emotions ranging from sadness to happiness, which in turn create a state of chronic dis-ease or vibrant health. Once you choose to move forward, take control, and make some positive changes, life becomes astonishing. There is no reason to sit back and *hope* that things will get better. Awareness allows you to see how you are presently living your life. Education offers you options to explore and change. Growth supports you in undertaking the options and reevaluating your journey.

Life can be hectic, especially with all of the responsibilities that people have to deal with on a daily basis. This drains us of our life force energy and leaves our minds unable to focus. Anxiety and other negative emotions arise, making it difficult to deal with people and our own mood swings. We are a society drowning in overdoses of medication and that has serious dysfunctional behavior with drugs, alcohol, smoking, etc. Our bodies are suffering, and we all look for a quick fix by taking a pill that will do more damage than good. We need to clear our blockages so we can become independent of prescription antidepressant, antianxiety, and sleeping medications. We have truly lost ourselves because our lives are moving at the speed of light. We are always rushing, multitasking, eating fast food, and not exercising or getting enough sunlight. Our energies are blocked on all levels, and we wonder why we feel tired, drained, ill, and cannot sleep.

Remember, every challenge you face can inspire necessary changes and movement forward. Change helps you to grow mentally, emotionally, and spiritually. Growth is not always easy, but it can chisel away at unwanted conditions. Welcome your growth with open arms. Look deep within yourself for answers. Become more aware of your lifestyle, your behavior, your motivations, and which aspects moved you toward the lifestyle you have chosen.

Once you begin your inner journey toward healing, spiritual growth and understanding will follow. Your consciousness and clarity will rise to new heights and continue to expand. Understanding your life's purpose and trusting your inner guidance bring a wonderful awareness within yourself. Your body, mind, and spirit open up, and you become whole. You become more understanding, caring, loving, forgiving, nonjudgmental, and *healthy*. Purpose becomes reality; you talk the talk and walk the walk. What an incredible feeling—loving yourself, feeling healthy, and being who you are meant to be.

We need more healers in this world so we can all live life in a more positive and healthy way. It is time for you to reclaim your energy, reclaim your power, and reclaim who you are! When you do, you will be more empowered than you have ever known yourself to be.

Part I

WHAT IS GENTLE ENERGY TOUCH?

Our bodies are more than just a collection of functioning parts and pieces. Just as we have a physical anatomy, we also have an energy anatomy. The human energy field called our aura surrounds and permeates the physical body. The goal of part 1 is to provide you with an in-depth understanding of the root cause of illness, the role our aura and seven major chakras play, and how to identify issues before they manifest as disease in the body. I will take you on a journey inside each of your seven chakras so you can understand what challenges it is time to let go of to heal yourself on all levels.

Every cell in our body works at either a high or low vibrational frequency. When the energy is low or blocked, we are more likely to get sick. When the energy is high, we can maintain our health and well-being. Though most people probably do not realize it, the majority of all physical disabilities and illnesses are triggered by negative energies that exist in the aura. Our aura is very sensitive to both positive and negative energy and allows both the positive and negative energy to cling to our physical body for years if left unchecked. When this happens, unhealthy behavioral patterns develop within the physical body that, over time, wear down the emotional, mental, and physical elements that make up that particular body. Part 1 teaches you how to cleanse and protect your aura and seven major chakras by practicing simple energy protection techniques.

Understand that as you begin your self-healing treatments, you may experience a cleansing period. The mind and body are being stimulated to release toxins, along with feelings and emotions that are no longer needed. Not only will you learn about the benefits of Gentle Energy Touch, auras, the seven major chakras, and energy protection, you will also come to understand the concept of prana energy and healing. Plus, you will learn how to experience feeling your own energy field—amazing! So let's begin, because there is a lot of information!

CHAPTER 1

The Basics

Gentle Energy Touch (GET) is a hands-on method that helps to create a feeling of inner peace. It shows you how to think of yourself as being lovable and grateful for what you already have. It enables you to explore and support your inner growth and spiritual development. It helps you take responsibility for your life and what you attract into it.

It is also a powerful technique that can relieve stress, encourage balance and harmony, and speed healing from traumas or injuries. It treats the whole person—the body, mind, and the spirit—in order to activate the healing process.

Gentle Energy Touch works on a wide array of conditions and produces long-lasting results. The categories below will give you a clear picture of how practicing this technique helps you.

Physical Benefits of Gentle Energy Touch

- Can be combined with other healing methods
- Assists you to take responsibility for your own healing
- Promotes the body's own natural ability to heal
- Helps release blocked energy associated with various issues such as smoking cessation, weight loss/weight gain, and other challenges

- Helps in restoring, healing, and balancing all seven major chakras
- Loosens blocked energy that could eventually cause disease
- Treats the root cause of illnesses
- Relieves pain—headaches, backaches, all sorts of pain—while relaxing the muscles
- Strengthens the immune system, allowing it to deal better with daily stress and anxiety
- Aids in a peaceful sleep when done an hour or two prior to bedtime
- Restores depleted energy and vitality
- Relaxes the body for aiding and improving fertility

Mental Benefits of Gentle Energy Touch

- Calms and relaxes the mind
- Promotes self-awareness so you can change your life for the better
- Improves the ability to concentrate by releasing blockages
- Helps to promote courage in making positive changes in one's life
- Promotes positive thinking and enhances meditation
- Removes the barriers that hold you back in life
- Creates inner harmony and awareness

Emotional Benefits of Gentle Energy Touch

- Helps to release fears
- Improves confidence and self-esteem
- Enhances relationships

- Promotes a deeper self-love and self-worth

- Assists in calming and balancing emotions

Spiritual Benefits of Gentle Energy Touch
- Does not conflict with religious beliefs

- Deepens connection with your Higher Self

- Increases intuition and other abilities

- Deepens fulfillment, self-realization, enlightenment, and Divine wisdom

GET and Ki

GET works by unblocking the natural flow of vital energy through the body. This vital energy or ki (also called chi or qi) continually courses through all living things and supports life. The vehicles through which this energy flows are called chakras. Also surrounding us is an energy field where ki is found; this is what's known as an aura. When ki gets stuck or blocked, we experience imbalance and illness. When ki flows freely and is in balance within the body, we have health and vitality.

All parts of our body, from our organs to our very cellular structure, are nourished and energized by ki. Ki is also directly related to positive thoughts (high vibration) or negative thoughts (low vibration), increasing or decreasing proportionally. When negative thoughts about ourselves lodge in our subconscious, they cause energy blockages, disrupting the flow of ki. Self-healing treatment allows the Universal Energy to respond to such disruptions and then go to that part of the body for healing.

As this greater energy flows through a person's energy field, that individual field gets charged with positive energy, thereby raising the vibratory level within the body. As a result, healing treatments clear the energy pathways of any blockages, increasing the flow of ki. The healing process can now proceed to any organs and cells that need it.

This healing energy can aid in repairing any kind of bodily distress such as heart disease, cancer, multiple sclerosis, skin problems, cuts and bruises, and a host of other challenges. *It is not in itself a cure, but it strengthens the body's natural defenses to release the root cause.*

This healing energy also works in harmony with all medical treatments or other healing modalities. It has been found that results from standard medical or psychological treatments improve when self-healing is practiced at the same time. Self-healing assists the body in healing at an accelerated rate by reducing the negative energy which has caused the medical condition in the first place or has accumulated from procedures such as surgery.

What you feel after a healing session can vary from person to person. Most often, you are left with a wonderfully relaxed, uplifted sensation. As you become more sensitive to the self-healing energy, you may experience fear, tension, anger, or even restlessness at certain hand position locations. This is usually an indication that the shadow side of an issue may be surfacing in your conscious or subconscious mind.

Regardless of what comes up, it is important to realize that as long as you are acknowledging the thoughts and experiencing the feelings, the treatment is effective. Issues that block energy flow appear so they can be released as the body prepares to complete the healing process. Observe without being judgmental and send love, light, and forgiveness to those issues.

Know that you are healed by your own intention to be well.

As you begin working with energy and with your self-healing positions, you may experience fluctuations in feelings or emotions as unresolved issues rise to the surface. These changes are part of the healing process and should be honored. Know that our body has its own wisdom. It sends us signals and messages and, many times, an illness or disease has an underlying symptom. It is very important that we find the root cause of the imbalance we are experiencing. Trust in your healing. All of this is an important part of the process of preparing if we plan to help others heal as well.

When Things Get Intense

If those changes are more intense than you feel able to handle, and life seems more difficult or troubled, you will find that saying positive affirmations can smooth the way as things eventually work out for a new and improved beginning. Concentrating on positive affirmations is calming, strengthening, and especially beneficial during self-healing and for sessions with a partner. Truly know that saying positive affirmations and allowing your body to relax will help you to heal physically, mentally, emotionally, and spiritually. I have included positive affirmations for your healing in appendix 1.

You'll also find links to three free sound files that I created especially for readers of this book in the Further Resources at the back of the book. The first contains a meditation to help you relax while you restore and rebalance your energy, the second meditation is to help you with self-confidence, and the third is to clear yourself of unwanted words and empower your potential.

When Not to Attempt a Healing

- It is important not to try a healing on someone else if you are sick or suffering from general weakness. You don't want to transfer your diseased energy to the person you are attempting to help!

- You should also not attempt a healing when you are feeling very angry, irritated, or judgmental, because the projected prana energy will be contaminated with that anger and other negative emotions. This may make the other person feel worse.

- You should not attempt a healing on someone if you think that person doubts your abilities or doesn't trust you in general.

- Never do a healing on someone if that person doesn't want it. Energy healing will not override a person's free will. The only time this does not apply is if someone is in a coma and unable to ask for healing. If you are doing healing on such a person or an infant or small child, always ask that individual's higher self for permission.

- Do not send healing energy to a broken bone because this may cause the bone to begin healing itself in an incorrect way. The bone must be set or put back in its place before healing is encouraged. Before the bone is set, you can do a sweep of the surrounding area with the intention to help remove pain, however. After the bone is set, then it is safe to apply healing energies.

- Do not send healing energy when someone is going for an x-ray, MRI, or any other type of procedure, including surgery. This may interfere with the outcome or results. Simply ask God or to whomever you pray to keep the person safe and to send their angels, loved ones, and spirit guides to watch over them. After the procedure and/or surgery, you can do healing on them if they ask.

CHAPTER 2

Your Seven Major Chakras

Since all healing depends on allowing the free flow of ki by opening the chakras, in this chapter we're going to take a rather deep dive into the chakras to explore what they are and how they work.

Let's start with the word itself, which derives from the ancient Sanskrit term meaning "spinning wheel of energy." These spinning wheels of energy receive, regulate, and disperse the vital life force energies within our bodies so we can function physically, mentally, emotionally, and spiritually. Within each chakra, the energy rotates like a turning wheel, functioning as a conduit for inflow and outflow.

Most literature—including this book—focuses on the seven major chakras, but we actually have hundreds of chakras all over the body. Each acupressure and acupuncture point is a chakra. When all the chakras are in harmony with an individual's consciousness, that person will be living as perfect a life as is possible on earth. However, very few people are so attuned that they can function perfectly aligned with all the chakras at the same time.

So how do chakras affect our bodies? Everything in the universe is composed of energy and vibrates at a particular frequency. This is true for both living beings and inanimate objects.

Our chakras can be pushed out of balance by all sorts of things. Just consider that all of the information and memories of your body's physical and conscious experiences are being stored in your chakras. What an intricate database! Every thought, every feeling, every memory you've ever had has been encoded and converted into matter, as a form of cellular memory. When these thoughts or memories are negative or traumatic, they can block the flow of energy in your body, draining vital life force energy from the chakras. The buildup of these negative messages and thoughts contributes to illness. As an example, issues of self-esteem belong to the third chakra (solar plexus) located at the lower chest and navel. Unresolved issues from childhood can block the energy and lead to health problems in this area.

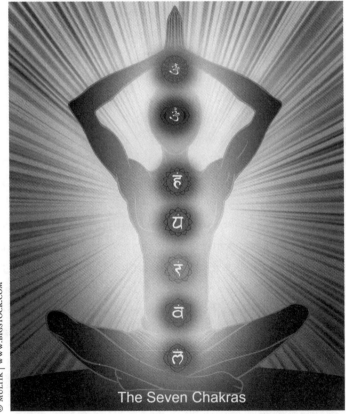

The Seven Chakras

© MULTIK | WWW.BIGSTOCK.COM

With chakra awareness we can also understand why we sometimes, for no explainable reason, fall ill when we are working hard to keep our body healthy. The way we act, think, and react to life's situations plays an important part in the manifestation of good and poor health in the various parts of the body.

I have found that we can best discover the underlying or root cause of a physical ailment simply by being aware of the chakras and their location. Lower back pain and difficulties handling money (hoarding or spending too much) can then be explained by lack of maturity in relationship development at the sacral chakra. Diabetes might correlate with low self-esteem or lack of personal control and a problem at the solar plexus chakra. Unresolved issues with our parents and physical problems are often connected with the root chakra. Discover the correlations of this powerful body map and the possibilities for healing unfold.

Let's now look at each chakra in turn.

The First Chakra, Root (Muladhara)

The first chakra, also known as the Security Center or Muladhara, is located at the base of the spine in the area of the tailbone. The root chakra is the foundation of our mental and emotional health. It filters energy up from the earth to our higher centers. It is at the root chakra that we connect to traditional beliefs and support the formation of our identity and a sense of belonging to a group. It is through this group or "tribal power" influence that lessons related to the material world are experienced.

The root chakra is associated with the color red and is responsible for producing this color in our energy field. The root chakra affects all the other chakras in a very powerful way. It steadily maintains a flow of solid energy, keeping our bodies grounded so we do not feel disoriented or scattered. Grounding keeps us balanced, down-to-earth, and connected with our physical body.

The root chakra is ready to send a spike of power up through all the other chakras whenever necessary, as long as they are not blocked and are able to respond. That means its effect on our vitality is crucial. Healing at this chakra improves our energy in general and brings us a new sense of well-being and balance.

A JOURNEY INTO THE FIRST CHAKRA

To understand and use this information, let's take a personal journey into the first chakra. Find a time to be quiet and a chair to sit comfortably in, while you breathe, relax, and form the intention to witness and explore what happens when you focus on one chakra at a time.

Physical Location: Base of spine in the area of the tailbone/coccyx

Feel the base of your spine where you are sitting, in the area of your tailbone. This is the physical location of the root chakra.

Color: Red

Next picture the color red streaming into this chakra. You can visualize this as a spotlight or a liquid stream of red entering your body at the site of this chakra. Take your time. Feel the vibration of this color. What are you feeling? What are you experiencing in this part of your body? Notice sensations, images, or anything that is happening to you in this moment. Do not judge what happens. Just be an observer.

Element: Earth

The root chakra represents earth. Let yourself feel magnetically connected to all of life. Feel your feet solidly planted on the floor. Feel yourself grounded and balanced.

Area of the Body Governed: Base of spine, legs, bones, feet, rectum, and immune system

Now feel how this part of your body connects with the rest of your body. Start with your feet. Feel how they connect to the floor. Let your awareness travel up your legs and then to your spine. Start at the base of your spine, next to your rectum, and let your awareness move up the rest of your spine. Now picture how your body protects itself: your immune system. This is a combination of systems involving your thymus gland, lymphatic system, and bone marrow. Let your consciousness flow through your body, picturing a strong, responsive immune system.

Qualities of a Grounded Root Chakra: Physical strength, health, patience, prosperity, security, vitality, and dynamic presence

Set your intention to focus on the qualities that this chakra represents. Take one quality at a time as you practice this meditation over a period of time and let yourself fully experience it. What does physical strength mean to you? How do you experience health? Ponder questions that allow you to focus and dwell on how these qualities appear, or do not appear, in your life. How can you enjoy these qualities in a balanced way?

Body System or Organ: Reproductive glands

Next bring your awareness to your reproductive organs and the glands that support them. Picture your reproductive organs and glands as healthy, vital, and alive. Combine this awareness with the sensation/vibration of the color red. Notice any sensations in this part of your body. Is the color red in this part of your body comfortable or not? How can you experience the power and glory of this part of your body? How do you connect with this sacred ground?

Physical Problems If Out of Balance: AIDS, Epstein-Barr virus, autoimmune diseases, arthritis, cancer, fatigue, and spinal and growth problems

Do you have any of the above dis-eases/conditions? How strong is your body? This is a time to focus on your health and the vitality that you want to experience. Do not judge your condition; let it teach you its lessons in order to improve your focus on your healing process. Picture yourself full of energy, enthusiasm, and enjoyment.

Information Stored in the Root Chakra: Family beliefs, super-stitions, loyalty, instincts, physical pleasure or pain, and touch

Go inside yourself; see if you have any "buttons" active with any of the above issues. Let this be a time of exploration, not judgment. Notice what your body tells you as you sit quietly and open your doors of perception.

Mental/Emotional Issues: Survival, self-esteem, social order, security, and family

This part of your body is about survival. How do you relate to your own survival? Are your basic needs met, or are you constantly struggling with money, food, housing, or other basic issues?

How do you feel about yourself? How is your self-esteem? Are you constantly critical of yourself? Can you enjoy being alone and bless the solitude?

Do you feel secure? What does this mean to you? Is security based on what you own, the talents you have, or on your ability to be flexible in any situation?

How do you relate to your family? Do you fit in? Are you seen as different, difficult, or strange? Some of us don't mesh with our families, although we can still love them dearly. Breaking away from the family rules can be a challenge, or it may be your norm.

How do you search for your identity? Is it tied to your family's definition, or are you searching for your own?

Underactive Root Issues: Unable to reach goals, lack of confidence, feeling unloved, not grounded, or feeling sexually inadequate

When the energy in this chakra is **underactive** or blocked, there can be issues to deal with. Do you have any problems with the qualities that are associated with this chakra being out of balance? This is a wonderful time to be honest with yourself and see how you can free yourself of qualities you no longer need or want.

Overactive Root Issues: Greed, egotism, bossiness, addiction to wealth, being high-strung, violent, dishonest, or cunning

When the energy in this chakra is **overactive** or blocked, there can be issues to deal with. Which of these qualities that are associated with this chakra do you have trouble with? This is a wonderful time to be open and honest with yourself and see how you can free yourself of qualities you no longer need or want.

Spiritual Lesson: Physical identity, material lessons, survival, or orientation on self-preservation

Now you have reached the spiritual level of lessons. How can you use the spiritual lessons of this chakra? How do they apply to you? Choose one of the lessons that reaches out to you, the one that speaks to you. Let yourself ponder it and see what happens inside you. Again, be a witness to the process. Explore and invite new possibilities for yourself.

Chakra Truth: We are All One, connected to all of life.

Every choice we make and every word we say influence the whole of life. Feel how you connect with life. Notice while you are sitting silently how you can blend with everything, become one with your breathing, with the surface you are sitting on, with the room you are in, with the city you are in, with the country, with the planet. Let this awareness grow, as you are ready to accept your part of the whole of life.

Our root chakra is the first on the chakra ladder and equivalent to the roots of a tree dug deep into the earth; it keeps us grounded. Without cleansing and healing this chakra, we become ungrounded, and—just like a tree with a weak attachment to the earth—the first real storm can topple us.

NOTES FOR THE FIRST CHAKRA

Focus on your health, the vitality that you want to experience.

Acknowledge and identify any fear you may have. Become aware of how you feel about it.

Replace it with the strength to overcome it. Build a solid foundation.

Trust in your healing.

The Second Chakra, Sacral (Svadhisthana)

The second chakra is known as the sacral chakra. It is located in the lower abdomen, encompassing the lower back and sex organs. The sacral chakra is the color orange. Its element is water. The sacral chakra is associated with the reproductive system, the pelvic area, the stimulation of our sexual desire, and our capacity for pleasure. It also energizes and balances those organs associated with the movement of fluid, such as the kidneys, urethra and bladder, the lymph system, and, to some extent, blood circulation. Its function is to keep everything moving and flowing.

A well-functioning sacral chakra maintains a healthy yin-yang and balanced existence. This allows for the coming together of our masculine and feminine sides as we develop spiritually, whether or not we have a partner. The masculine side deals with such things as action, logic, organization, ambition, and drive and is governed by the left-brain. The feminine side deals with such things as verbal skills, creativity, musical and artistic abilities and is governed by the right-brain. Development of the sacral chakra moves us toward internal balance between our driving and nurturing principles.

Power plays and security issues are associated with the sacral chakra. This chakra offers us the opportunity to reduce our "control issues" and find balance in our lives. A healthy sacral chakra teaches us to recognize that acceptance and rejection are not the only options in our relationships.

The sacral chakra is where we begin to process emotions and look outward toward having a relationship with others. We begin to expand, grow, and move beyond ourselves. We begin connecting to other individuals through feelings, desire, sensation, and movement. At the root chakra, the focus was primarily on our inner self. Here at the sacral chakra, we start to look outward at our connections to the world. We begin embracing these ties. We focus on our social life on a personal level with friends, lovers, and family and in a broader sense within a global community.

It is here at the sacral chakra that we begin to feel sexual intimacy. The sacral is the center for nurturing and tenderness. It prompts us to take care of ourselves and to take care of others. It allows us to enjoy both the giving and receiving of sensual (not necessarily sexual) pleasure. The need for touch and nurturing is as basic as the need for food and water. Touch becomes a major form of communication, whether as parents cuddling our children, strangers meeting with a handshake, friends giving affection, or as lovers giving sexual pleasure.

With a healthy sacral chakra, we begin to enjoy touching as well as being touched. We begin to understand about giving as well as receiving. In sexual relationships, we develop from taking what we want to giving as part of being intimate. Sex becomes more than a mere biological function; it now includes sexual intimacy as a form of communication and mutual comfort. The focus shifts from "me" to "us," and the desire to please becomes a major part of the equation. Here we refine sex and lust to become desire and love.

Men and woman experience sexual intimacy and desire quite differently. Women tend to tap into a deep sense of affection and commitment associated with their sexuality. Men are more governed by their physical desires. Men usually take longer to develop a sense of intimacy and commitment.

When two people find each other sexually attractive and fall in love, the sacral chakra opens. When the heart chakra that deals with human loving and the throat chakra that governs ideas and communication also open, suddenly there is this connection that causes creativity and inspiration in a tremendously exciting way.

After the initial opening, the sacral chakra begins to balance, and the level of sexual activity and the mood also begin to stabilize. This allows a return to normal everyday activity while the connection between the couple remains strong.

When two people who are open at the sacral level come together, there's often an accompanying sense of having known each other before and of being meant to be together. Thus, a mutually satisfying and healthy relationship is formed.

This chakra has to do with the balance and smooth flowing of energy within us and with others. Blockage at this level can manifest itself in a fear of being controlled. Loss of control, reluctance to take risks, feeling abandoned by others, having a sense of loss of personal identity through such events as assault, feeling guilty, blaming others, being unable to maintain close relationships or ending them prematurely for fear of rejection can manifest as well.

Areas of potential issues identified with the sacral chakra are risk-taking, money, power, creativity, decision-making, rebelliousness, and ethics.

Physical manifestations with a blocked sacral chakra include but are not limited to uterine illness/endometriosis, fibroids, ovarian cysts, tumors, menopause difficulties, urinary problems and prostate difficulties, lower back and hip pain, and arthritis.

Balance in the sacral chakra is vital to our successful functioning and survival in society and can insure peace, harmony, health, and satisfying relationships throughout our lifetime.

A JOURNEY INTO THE SECOND CHAKRA

To understand and use this general information, let's take a personal journey into the second chakra—our sacral chakra. Find a time to be quiet and sit comfortably, while you breathe, relax, and set the intention to witness and explore what happens when you focus on this chakra.

Physical Location: Lower abdomen to the navel

Feel your lower back and abdomen up to your navel, including your sexual organs. This is the physical location of the sacral chakra. Let your mind focus on this part of your body.

Color: Orange

Next picture the color orange streaming into this chakra. You can visualize this as a spotlight or a liquid stream of orange entering your body at the site of this chakra. Take your time. Sense the vibration of this color. What are you feeling? What are you experiencing in this part of your body? Notice sensations, images, or anything that is happening to you at this moment. Do not judge what happens. Just be an observer.

Element: Water

Let yourself feel how water flows. Our body is more than 60 percent water. It is an element that cleanses when it is flowing and able to move freely. When it is not flowing or blocked in some way, it stagnates and becomes polluted. This is a time to feel the "waters" in your body flowing. These "waters" can include your blood, saliva, tears, and other bodily fluids.

Area of the Body Governed: Lower abdomen to naval, sexual organs, large intestine, lower vertebrae of your spine, pelvis, appendix, kidneys, bladder, and hip area

Now focus on your lower abdomen, the area where your sexual organs are located. Let your awareness expand to your lower back, around to the front of your abdomen and then to your navel. Allow yourself to go deep inside your body, to your intestines and your kidneys, and imagine taking a journey inside your body. Explore what this part of your body is about for you. Enjoy the journey.

Qualities of the Sacral Chakra: Shows concern for others, creative, friendly, good-humored, sexual satisfaction, balanced, desire for pleasure, prosperity, and procreation

Set your intention to focus on the qualities that this chakra represents. Take one quality at a time and let yourself fully experience each one. What does "concern for others" mean to you? How do you experience creativity? Ask yourself questions that allow you to focus and dwell on how these qualities appear, or do not appear, in your life. How can you enjoy these qualities in a balanced way?

Body System or Organ: Genitourinary tract

Next bring your awareness to your genitals and urinary organs. Picture your kidneys and reproductive organs as healthy, vital, and alive. Combine this awareness with the sensation/vibration of the color orange. Notice any sensations in this part of your body. Is the color orange in this part of your body comfortable or not? How can you experience the power and glory of this part of your body? How do you connect with this "sacral" ground?

Physical Problems If Out of Balance: Uterine problems, endometriosis, fibroids, ovarian cysts, tumors, menopause difficulties, fertility problems, urinary and prostate difficulties, back and hip pain, and arthritis

Do you have any of the above dis-eases/conditions? How strong is your body? This is a time to focus on your health and the vitality that you want to experience. Picture yourself full of energy, enthusiasm, and enjoyment. Do not judge your condition. Be aware of the lessons this chakra has to teach. Focus on your healing process in this area.

Information Stored in the Sacral Chakra: Duality, magnetism, controlling patterns, and emotional feelings such as joy, anger, and fear

Go inside yourself, and see if you have any "buttons" active with any of the above issues. You may experience sensations of pleasure or pain. Let this be a time of exploration, not judgment. Focus on what your body tells you as you sit quietly. Open your doors of perception.

Mental/Emotional Issues: Blame, guilt, money concerns, sex, power, control, creativity, and morality

This part of your body holds the above mental issues. Do you have problems with blame or guilt? What are your thoughts about touch, being touched, and your sexuality? How do you relate to your sexuality? How does your sexuality relate to your need to control, your sense of power, or your spirituality? Take the time to be open and honest with yourself.

Underactive Sacral Issues: Shy, hides emotions, timid, overly sensitive, guilt feelings, distrustful

When the energy in this chakra is **underactive** or blocked, there can be issues to deal with. Do you have problems with the qualities that are associated with this chakra being out of balance? This is a wonderful time to be open and honest with yourself and see how you can set yourself free of the qualities you no longer need or want.

Overactive Sacral Issues: Explosive, aggressive, self-serving, manipulative, arrogant, high-strung, selfish, lustful, and conceited

When the energy in this chakra is **overactive** or blocked, there can be issues to deal with. Which of these qualities that are associated with this chakra do you have trouble with? This is a wonderful time to be open and honest with yourself and see how you can free yourself of qualities you no longer need or want.

Spiritual Lesson: Creativity, manifestation, honoring relationships and learning to let go, ability to access key childhood experiences

How can you grow from the spiritual lessons of this chakra? How do they apply to you? This chakra has many lessons. Choose one that reaches out to you, the one that speaks to you. Let yourself ponder this and see what happens inside you. Again, be a witness to the process. Explore and invite new possibilities for yourself.

Chakra Truth: Honor one another and ourselves with truth. Every relationship you develop helps you become more conscious in encouraging love and harmony with others.

In focusing on the truth of this chakra, you have an opportunity to first honor yourself. What does this mean to you? As you learn to honor yourself, you then can start to honor another. How do you create peace and harmony inside yourself? In turn, how can you become more conscious to insure peace and harmony with others? Union implies relationship.

What value do your relationships have? How are you growing spiritually from these relationships?

NOTES FOR THE SECOND CHAKRA

Acknowledge and identify your relationships with work, money, creativity, friends, and family. Become aware of how you feel about these relationships.

Are you afraid of change?

Trust in your healing.

The Third Chakra, Solar Plexus (Manipura)

The solar plexus is where our willpower and the ability to make things happen are located. This is the area that defines our self-esteem, confidence, self-worth, and personality. This is where we learn to maintain strong boundaries and a personal code of honor. The personality that develops during our teenage years is in this chakra, otherwise called "ego." Anyone experiencing dysfunction of the solar plexus chakra is having difficulty obtaining or maintaining their "personal power." This intuitive chakra is where we find our "gut instinct"—the signal to do or not to do something without knowing why. A strong sense of self-esteem is required for developing intuitive skills.

The solar plexus chakra occupies the area between the lower chest and navel and is associated with the color yellow. Here we find passion and energy, filled with opinion, logic, motivation, and drive. This is the chakra of our personal power; it gives us the choice to create our own life strategy in whatever way we wish. The solar plexus offers us freedom. Opinions are born from this area. It is here that we develop the courage to express ourselves in the world. We discover our inner strength and freedom in order to keep going despite any difficult life events.

A balanced solar plexus offers us unlimited possibilities: to work, create change, to become what we want to be, to realize our ambitions and be happy, to steer our lives in any direction. We learn to accept responsibility for ourselves and our choices.

With the opening of the solar plexus and development of self-esteem comes a growing ability to respect others for who they are. We appreciate change as a gift and see it as a challenge that helps us grow. We learn to adapt, accommodate differences, and refine our opinions and beliefs. We become willing to compromise to ensure easy progress and development.

However, problems with the development of our personality and personal power can manifest themselves in many ways. Those who have issues in the solar plexus chakra may find it difficult to handle crises, accept criticism, or express self-confidence; they feel fearful and mistrusting. Also, medically speaking, areas within the middle abdomen may become diseased and can manifest as hepatitis, cirrhosis, diabetes, colitis, cholecystitis, hiatal hernia, and ulcers. The solar plexus is also connected to the digestive system and to physical assimilation of food and nutrients.

Proper functioning of the solar plexus chakra enables us to live an empowered, respectable life with a sense of courage and inner strength. The amazing force produced by a combination of power and will makes us capable of more than we ever imagined. When we add the greatest power of all—love—wonderful things happen.

A JOURNEY INTO THE THIRD CHAKRA

To better understand and use this information, let's explore the aspects of the third chakra—our solar plexus. Find a time to be quiet and sit comfortably, while you breathe, relax, and set the intention to witness and explore what happens when you focus on this chakra.

Physical Location: Solar plexus (mid-abdomen between lower chest and navel)

Feel your solar plexus between your lower chest and navel. This is the physical location of this chakra. Let your mind focus on this part of your body.

Color: Yellow

Next picture the color yellow streaming into this chakra. You can visualize this as a spotlight or a liquid stream of yellow entering your body at this chakra. Take your time. Feel the vibration of this color. What do you sense? What are you experiencing in this part of your body? Notice sensations, images, or anything that is happening to you in this moment. Do not judge what happens. Just be an observer.

Element: Fire

Your body has several areas that can be considered centers that generate or regulate heat. Perspiration is one example of how we regulate the heat or fire of the body. Three systems relate closely to how much fire is in the body: the circulatory system, respiratory system, and sexual organs. Take this time to look inside your body to feel where you are sensitive to heat or find an internal fire.

Area of the Body Governed: Muscular system, abdomen, stomach, small and large intestines, liver, gallbladder, kidneys, pancreas, adrenal glands, spleen, middle spine

Take a deep breath in and, as you exhale, focus on your middle abdomen; feel how this part of your body connects with the rest of your body. Stretch your arms out, stretch your legs, feel your entire body. Feel the strength in your abdomen, feel the strength in your bones and muscular system, and feel the strength of all the areas governed by the solar plexus. Ask yourself this question: "Do I take care of my body or do I abuse it?" Let your consciousness flow through your body, picturing a healthy system.

Qualities of the Solar Plexus Chakra: Outgoing, cheerful, respect for oneself and others, skillful, spontaneous, open and expressive, intelligent, self-confident, flexible, decisive, vitality, effectiveness, spontaneity, and nondominating

Set your intention to focus on the qualities that this chakra represents. How can you enjoy these qualities in a balanced way? Can you be flexible in a situation? How spontaneous are you? Do you have energy to spare or do you feel drained? See how you can experience the above qualities fully in your daily life.

Body System or Organ: Pancreas

Next bring your awareness to your pancreas, located horizontally across the upper abdomen. Picture this part of your body as healthy, vital, and alive. Combine this awareness with the sensation/vibration of the color yellow. Notice any sensations in this part of your body. Is the color yellow in this part of your body comfortable or not? How can you experience the sweetness of this part of your body?

Physical Problems If Out of Balance: Hepatitis, cirrhosis, diabetes, colitis, cholecystitis, hiatal hernia, and ulcers

The solar plexus is also connected to the digestive system and to physical assimilation of food and nutrients. Do you have any of the above dis-eases/conditions? How strong is your body? This is a time to focus on your health and the vitality that you want to experience. Picture yourself full of energy, enthusiasm, and enjoyment. Do not judge your condition; let it teach you the lessons it has to improve your focus on your healing process.

Information Stored in the Solar Plexus Chakra: Personal power, personality, consciousness of self within the universe, sense of belonging and knowing

Go inside yourself, and see if you have any "buttons" active with any of the above issues. Is personal power a goal for you? Do you feel a sense of belonging in your body? How do you sense a feeling of just knowing things? These are issues to dwell on while you listen to the answers that come from within.

Mental/Emotional Issues: Trust, fear, intimidation, self-esteem, self-confidence, self-respect, ambition, courage, ability to handle crises, care of yourself and others, sensitivity to criticism, personal honor, fear of rejection and looking foolish, physical appearance anxieties, and strength of character

When you trust the universe, all is well. When you experience your life through the eyes of fear, the world seems a bleak place indeed. It is all about choice. How do you choose to think about a particular situation? Make time today to focus on the positive mental side of this chakra. How can you turn fear into love? How can you trust that the universe is here to support you? In what way do you express your strength of character? How do you care for yourself and, in turn, others?

Find thoughts that support you to operate with trust, to experience love in your life, and to care for yourself with joy. As you do this, your sensitivity to criticism will lessen and you will learn that most criticism comes from the other person's unresolved issues. Personal honor can be experienced every day.

Underactive Solar Plexus Issues: Lack of self, blame for others, depression, feeling isolated and deprived of recognition, fear of failure, poor judgment, apathy, confused

When the energy in this chakra is **underactive** or blocked, there can be issues to deal with. Do you have problems with the qualities that are associated with this chakra being out of balance? This is a wonderful time to see how you can free yourself of qualities you no longer need or want.

Overactive Solar Plexus Issues: Very demanding, being a workaholic, judgmental, perfectionist, critical, always planning but never manifesting, and stubbornness

When the energy in this chakra is **overactive** or blocked, there can be issues to deal with. Do you have problems with the qualities that are associated with this chakra being out of balance? This is a wonderful time to be honest with yourself and see how you can free yourself of qualities you no longer need or want.

Spiritual Lesson: Acceptance of your place in the life stream, human and Divine love

How can you use the spiritual lessons of this chakra? How do they apply to you? This chakra has deep lessons. How do you accept your place in the stream of life? How do you experience human love, Divine love? Let yourself ponder these questions and see what happens inside you. Again, be a witness to the process. Explore and invite new possibilities for yourself.

Chakra Truth: Accept responsibility for the person you have become.

How can you honor the relationship you have with yourself? How do you accept responsibility for the person you have become? These are issues that affect our very core. Honoring the relationship you have with yourself may mean taking a nap when you are tired instead of pushing through, for example.

Accepting responsibility for the person you have become might mean looking at how you respond in certain situations. Is your first response one of anger or aggravation, or is it one of understanding and joy? Learning the sacred truth about yourself in relation to this chakra is something that can be done daily and can bring about lovely changes in you as an individual with personal character. Embrace the challenge, and see how you relate to this sacred truth.

NOTES FOR THE THIRD CHAKRA

Acknowledge and identify how your self-esteem is. Are you feeling strong or frightened?

Do you need someone's approval? Are you judgmental or critical of yourself or others?

Are you courageous?

Trust in your healing.

The Fourth Chakra, Heart (Anahata)

The heart chakra is the center of the entire human energy system. This chakra is associated with the color green and/or pink. The purpose of this center is to achieve perfect union through love, and it is often the focus in bringing about healing. The words "love heals all" hold a great truth. "Love" is the energy of a healthy heart chakra. The feelings of love that we experience between lovers, friends, parents, children, or pets are all the same energies.

Situations such as divorce or separation, death of a loved one, abuse, abandonment, or adultery are all wounding to the heart chakra and can cause deep emotional problems. Physical illness brought about by heartbreak requires that an emotional healing occur along with the physical healing. Since air is the element of this chakra, time spent each day sitting quietly and meditating on your breath will be richly rewarded by improvements in your immune system. From its location in the middle of the chest, the heart chakra radiates its healing energy to the farthest point of our being and into the energetic atmosphere. Without the proper functioning of this one chakra, we cease to exist as human beings. It is in this chakra that love, compassion, and touch reside.

When our heart chakra opens, it influences us to reassess our relationship with ourselves and our connection with everything else in the universe. This chakra is the bridge in our spiritual ascent, bringing together the lower and upper three chakras. The first three chakras hold us securely in our human state, while chakras five, six, and seven above guide us toward the spiritual. When we hold grudges or wish to seek revenge, act jealous of someone or their possessions, and are unable to trust others, then growth in this area is stunted. This can lead to the obvious illnesses such as heart attack, angina, and congestive heart failure, as well as asthma, emphysema, lung or breast cancer, bronchitis, and esophagitis. "Letting go" and "moving on" enable us to resolve issues. When we begin to love selflessly and have a "healthy heart," a well-functioning fourth chakra enables all the other chakras, transforming us into a channel for Divine love. Our essence radiates natural warmth, sincerity, happiness, confidence, joy, compassion, but most of all love.

A JOURNEY INTO THE FOURTH CHAKRA

To understand and use this information, let's take a personal journey into this fourth chakra—our heart chakra. Find a time to be quiet and sit comfortably, while you breathe, relax, and set the intention to witness and explore what happens when you focus on this chakra.

Physical Location: Center of the chest

Feel the center of your chest. The organ of your heart is actually on your left side, under your breastbone. Let your mind focus on this part of your body. Feel the beat of your heart.

Color: Green and secondary color pink

Next picture the color green and/or pink streaming into this chakra. You can visualize this as a spotlight or a liquid stream of green entering your body at the site of this chakra. Take your time. Feel the vibration of this color. What do you feel? What are you experiencing in this part of your body? Notice sensations, images, or anything that is happening to you in this moment. Do not judge what happens. Just be an observer.

Element: Air

This element can be understood as the air we breathe or the breath itself. This is the perfect time to focus on your breath. A simple meditation is to focus on the air coming into your nose. Are you breathing more into your left or right nostril? As the air comes in, let your attention go to your throat. Feel the breath going down as you inhale and coming back out of your throat as you exhale. Let your attention go farther down into your rib cage to your lungs. Feel them expand and contract as you breathe in and out. Let your focus go to your diaphragm, at the base of your lungs. As you inhale, you can let your belly expand, feeling it as low as your sacrum. As you exhale, notice if you can let your belly and lower back contract gently. This simple meditation can take as long as you wish. It is both relaxing and informative. Notice which parts of your body are easy to sense.

Area of the Body Governed: Heart, circulatory system, blood, lungs, rib cage, diaphragm, thymus, breasts, esophagus, shoulders, arms, and hands

Now focus on your rib cage. Feel how this part of your body connects with the rest of your body. It is possible to measure your pulse in many places throughout your body. Find one of these spots and focus on how your circulatory system speaks to you. Our hands map out our body. Treat your body by massaging your hands or feet. Spend a few minutes massaging one hand with the other. Notice what you feel. Touching and loving yourself is what the heart chakra is all about.

Qualities of the Heart Chakra: Love, compassion, peacefulness, centeredness, and spirituality

Set your intention to focus on the qualities that this chakra represents. How can you enjoy these qualities in a balanced way? One thought to repeat is, "May I feel centered and peaceful." Or you can substitute another quality that speaks to you, such as, "May I feel compassion and love for myself and others." Make up sentences that suit your needs, and repeat these throughout the day, substituting negative thoughts for positive loving ones.

Body System or Organ: Thymus gland, controlling the immune system

Next bring your awareness to your chest. The thymus gland is in your upper chest, below your throat. Combine this awareness with the sensation/vibration of the color green or pink. Notice any sensations in this part of your body. Is the color green or pink in this part of your body comfortable or not? Tapping this part of your body stimulates your immune system. Gently tap or thump your thymus with your fingertips (about twenty times) and feel the sensation travel throughout your body.

Physical Problems If Out of Balance: Heart attack, angina, congestive heart failure, as well as asthma, AIDS, emphysema, lung or breast cancer, bronchitis, carpal tunnel syndrome
Do you have any of the above dis-eases/conditions? How strong is your body? This is a time to focus on your health and the vitality that you want to experience. Picture yourself full of energy, enthusiasm, and enjoyment. Do not judge your condition; let it teach you the lessons it has to improve your focus on your healing process.

Information Stored in the Heart Chakra: Connections or "heartstrings" to those whom we love
Go inside yourself and picture the people you love. Even better, picture those you do not get along with, those you have closed your heart to. This is an opportunity to open your heart and be nice to those who challenge your feelings. Send love to these individuals. Forgive them and forgive yourself and move on with your life.

Mental/Emotional Issues: Love, hatred, bitterness, grief, anger, jealousy, inability to forgive, self-centeredness, fear of loneliness, commitment and betrayal, compassion, hope, and trust
When you experience love or hate, you are feeling emotions that can sometimes seem out of control. This is your chance to examine how the contradictory emotions above can come into better

balance inside yourself. What do you feel bitter about? Are their areas of grief you have not resolved? Where does anger or jealousy limit your ability to feel love? Do you experience a fear of loneliness? Can you open your heart and let hope and trust blossom?

Underactive Heart Issues: Self-pity, afraid of letting go and getting hurt, paranoia, need for reassurance, indecisiveness, uncertainty and unable to enforce will, and feeling unloved

When the energy in this chakra is **underactive** or blocked, there can be issues to deal with. Do you have issues with the qualities that are associated with this chakra being out of balance? This is a wonderful time to see how you can free yourself of qualities you no longer need or want.

Overactive Heart Issues: Being overly critical, possessive, jealous, blaming others, demanding, angry, an attitude of coldness, self-doubt, and mistrustfulness

When the energy in this chakra is **overactive** or blocked, there can be issues to deal with. Do you have problems with the qualities that are associated with this chakra being out of balance? This is a wonderful time to be honest with yourself and see how you can free yourself of qualities you no longer need or want.

Spiritual Lesson: Forgiveness, unconditional love, letting go, compassion, and trust

How can you use the spiritual lessons of this chakra? How do they apply to you? Understanding how to forgive is really a gift to yourself. It is as if, in our anger, we take poison and hope the other person dies from it. Let yourself ponder how compassion and letting go can open your heart. When you have compassion for yourself, it is easier to be compassionate to others. This allows you to feel trust in the universe and how it can and does support you. Explore and invite new possibilities for yourself.

Chakra Truth: See the beauty in everyone and everything. Love and forgiveness are the true motivators of our body, mind, and spirit.

When we spend our emotional energy on anger or hate, we squander one of our most precious resources. When we see the beauty in ourselves, in others, in everyone and everything, we open our heart to the sacred truth that love is the supreme source of energy. Love can become our motivator, healing our body and uniting our mind and spirit.

NOTES FOR THE FOURTH CHAKRA

Acknowledge and identify whom you need to forgive.

Are you feeling love, bitterness, or hurt feelings from your heart?

Is your heart full of anger? Send out love and forgive.

Trust in your healing.

What have you learned about yourself up to this point?

Write down at least five changes you have noticed and what significance these have in your life.

The Fifth Chakra, Throat (Vishuddha)

The fifth chakra, the throat chakra, is the center of expression, communication, and inspiration. It is here at this chakra that we express what we think, feel, see, and desire. With vision, thought, knowledge, and understanding, this chakra connects us to our world and enables us to receive and assimilate information. This information is then used to communicate the contents of all the chakras through verbal expression.

The throat chakra also connects our "intellectual self" to our "feeling self." It is the throat that allows us to express verbally what we have only learned to feel. Through this chakra we say yes or no to life's options, for it is the link between emotion and thought.

The Sanskrit name for the throat chakra is "Vishuddha," which means pure. The healthfulness of the throat chakra relates to how honestly we express ourselves. Not speaking or coming from truth violates our body and our spirit.

All choices we make in our lives have consequences on an energetic level. Even choosing not to make a choice, such as repressing our anger, may manifest into laryngitis. We have all experienced that "lump in our throats" when we don't know how to voice the right words. Often, we tend to speak carelessly and without thought or consideration. However, as we recognize the consequences of spoken words, we learn to choose them more wisely and carefully. Once released into the universe, they can never be retrieved.

One benefit of an opened throat chakra is telepathy. We are all gifted with this skill to some extent, particularly with people we love or are in tune with. Most mothers, even from a great distance, can tune in to their children and feel when something is wrong. Most of us have experienced getting ready to phone someone but they phone us first. An evolved throat chakra makes telepathy possible. How is this communication accomplished? The medium for these thoughts is the energetic atmosphere, called the ether, which is the element of the throat chakra. It is a subtle heavenly energy and a unifying field from which all particles, all matter, and all things physical arise. There is no space between us, since in the final analysis, we are all joined in spirit.

When we have loving thoughts of a family member for example, the vibrations of those thoughts go into the atmosphere and to their target. Even if the person doesn't realize that love is being sent, that person's life will be enhanced anyway. Conversely, sending hateful thoughts can cause damage to someone. Since everything will come back to us eventually, we need to make sure that what we send out is with love for the higher good of the person concerned.

The throat chakra's color is bright blue. This chakra connects the neck, the throat, vocal cords, the thyroid and parathyroid glands, the mouth, trachea, esophagus, ears, and cervical spine. When the throat chakra is blocked or sluggish, it will often manifest physically in recurrent sore throats, colds, swollen glands, neck pains, and dental problems. There may be symptoms of hypothyroidism with lethargy, weight gain, low mood, or coarsening of the skin and hair. Symptoms of hyperthyroidism may include weight loss, anxiety, poor sleep, and increased energy with jitteriness. Throat cancer or even being mute may be present.

Communication is essential to our existence. A free flow of energy in the throat chakra is imperative to allow us personal expression and the ability to make decisions and to follow our dreams.

A JOURNEY INTO THE FIFTH CHAKRA

To understand and use this information, let's take a personal journey into this fifth chakra—our throat chakra. Find a time to be quiet and sit comfortably, while you breathe, relax, and set the intention to witness and explore what happens when you focus on this chakra.

Physical Location: Throat and neck region

Feel your neck and throat. Make easy circles with your head, first in one direction, then in the opposite, letting your neck and throat rotate and release the tension we tend to store here. Let your mind focus on this part of your body.

Color: Blue

Next picture the color blue streaming into this chakra. You can visualize this as a spotlight or a liquid stream of blue entering your body at the site of this chakra. Take your time. Sense the vibration of this color. What do you feel? What are you experiencing in this part of your body? Notice sensations, images, or anything that is happening to you in this moment. Do not judge what happens. Just be an observer.

Element: Sound

Our throat is the epicenter for sound. Sounds can be so healing. Explore making sounds of all kinds: loud/soft, move the sound from the front of your throat to the back, animal noises, grunts, groans, moans, sighs, musical notes, or whatever you want to make up at the time. Have fun making sounds. Notice how you feel afterwards. Stimulated? More awake? Soothed?

Area of the Body Governed: Throat, thyroid gland, parathyroid gland, trachea, neck, cervical vertebrae, mouth, teeth, gums, and esophagus

Now focus on your throat, your neck, your mouth, your teeth and gums, and feel how your neck and throat connect your head to the rest of your body.

Qualities of the Throat Chakra: Balanced energy, clear communication, creativity, manifesting in the physical world the fulfillment of one's goals, sincerity, independence, truthfulness, and living in the present

Set your intention to focus on the qualities that this chakra represents. How can you enjoy these qualities in a balanced way? What does living in the present mean to you? Can you focus on *now*—not the past or the future, but *now?* Picture yourself filled with balanced, clear energy. Hear yourself communicating clearly—expressing your creativity, your independence, and your sincerity. This is a good time to write down your goals. What would you like to see yourself doing with the healing information you are learning here?

Body System or Organ: Thyroid gland

Next bring your awareness to the base of your throat. This is where your thyroid gland is located. Picture this part of your body as healthy, vital, and alive. Combine this awareness with the sensation/vibration of the color blue. Notice any sensations in this part of your body. Is the color blue in this part of your body comfortable or not? How can you express yourself clearly with your words, your sounds?

Physical Problems If Out of Balance: Sore throat, inflammation, burns, skin irritations, fever, ear infections, overtiredness, mental exhaustion, gum inflammations, esophagitis, nervousness, back pain, hemorrhoids, high blood pressure, weight gain, low mood, weight loss, anxiety, poor sleep, throat cancer, mutism

Do you have any of the above dis-eases/conditions? How strong is your body? This is a time to focus on your health and the vitality that you want to experience. Picture yourself full of energy, enthusiasm, and enjoyment. Do not judge your condition; let it teach you the lessons it has to improve your focus on your healing process.

Information Stored in the Throat Chakra: Self-knowledge, truth, attitudes, hearing, taste, and smell

Go inside yourself and see if you have any "buttons" active with any of the above issues. What helps you to hear what you need, to hear the truth, to hear attitude—yours or someone else's?

Mental/Emotional Issues: Personal expression, creativity, addiction, criticism, faith, decision-making, will, and lack of authority

Do you have addictions? They can be simple ones like being addicted to watching television every night, or they can be chemical in nature—smoking, drinking, or sugar consumption. What are you willing to do to give up these habits—especially the harmful ones? Do you take criticism well or not so well? Do you say what you need to with honesty or exaggerate to make others like you? Are you comfortable with taking charge, expressing your will, or making decisions? This is a time for self-reflection. Listen to the voices inside your head. Listen to your heart. Is there a difference?

Underactive Throat Issues: Surrenders to others, slow to respond, resists change, melancholy, stubborn

When the energy in this chakra is **underactive** or blocked, there can be issues to deal with. Do you have problems with the qualities that are associated with this chakra being out of balance? This is a wonderful time to see how you can free yourself of qualities you no longer need or want.

Overactive Throat Issues: Domineering, dogmatic, overreacting, speaks negatively/harshly, clings to tradition, hyperactive

When the energy in this chakra is **overactive** or blocked, there can be issues to deal with. Do you have problems with the qualities that are associated with this chakra being out of balance? This is a wonderful time to be honest with yourself and see how you can free yourself of qualities you no longer need or want.

Spiritual Lesson: Confession, surrender personal will to Divine will, faith and truthfulness over deceit

How can you use the spiritual lessons of this chakra? How do they apply to you? Are you willing to express truth, your truth, as well as listen to Divine will? What is God's plan for you? How can you stop deceiving yourself and others? Are you willing to feel the link between your emotions and your thinking? This chakra has many lessons. Now you have reached the spiritual level of lessons. Choose one of the lessons that reaches out to you, the one that speaks to you. Let yourself ponder this and see what happens inside you. Again, be a witness to the process. Explore and invite new possibilities for yourself.

Chakra Truth: Choice and strength. Having the insight and faith to surrender personal will to Divine will. Every action and thought we create has global consequences.

When you surrender your will to Divine will, your life will take a huge turn. It is like stepping off a cliff and not putting a safety net underneath us. And yet if you take that step knowing that you are supported by Divine love and guidance, you can start to live your life with actions motivated by a personal will that trusts Divine authority, which can give your life a richness you can scarcely imagine. Take that step, knowing you are safe.

NOTES FOR THE FIFTH CHAKRA

Acknowledge and identify your needs and desires.

Are you feeling drained by the choices you made today?

Is your communication with others honest and with integrity?

Trust in your healing.

The Sixth Chakra, Brow or Third Eye (Ajna)

The sixth chakra, whose Sanskrit name is "Ajna," is where we ultimately take command of our lives. This chakra is called the consciousness awareness center for the entire mind, body, and spirit. With the awakening of this chakra, we find inspiration, perception, and vision.

The brow chakra, often called the "third eye," is associated with the color indigo or midnight blue and is located above and between the eyes. It is the center of intuition and reasoning. It is our avenue to wisdom—our learning from experiences and putting them in perspective. This chakra allows us to separate reality from fantasy. It is through an open brow chakra that visual images are received.

At the sixth chakra, we see beyond physical seeing, hear beyond human hearing, and use intuition beyond rational explanation. This chakra allows seeing in the deeper sense of inner vision and intuition.

On the spiritual level, the brow chakra governs our sixth sense of awareness. It is here that we can receive guidance and tune in to our higher self. The third eye opens us up to other senses like clairvoyance and clairaudience. The former is the ability to see into the future, while the latter is the ability to hear spirit voices and other vibration frequencies not sensed by the human ear. The brow chakra brings all the other chakras together where our spirituality may finally reach full bloom.

On a physical level, this chakra governs the pituitary gland, skull, eyes, brain, and nervous system. It regulates many of our hormonal and endocrine functions. Our endocrine glands have an effect on the body from cellular gene activation to the functioning of the central nervous system. Therefore, this chakra is able to affect our behavior and moods through hormonal influences on brain activity. The pituitary glands, the nervous system, and the brain control the messages sent to the rest of the body. The skull protects the brain from outside interference, and the eyes allow us to see on the physical level. This chakra also governs our five senses.

If the brow chakra is unbalanced, our physical state of existence can become nonassertive; we can become afraid of success or go the opposite way and be egotistical. Sickness will then manifest in the way we think. If the energy from our brain and pituitary does not flow in a positive and balanced direction, we may suffer many types of ailments such as headaches, sinus and nasal problems, blurred vision, blindness, eyestrain, and disease within the brain and skull.

When the brain waves that govern our emotions are disoriented with negative thinking, they can cause us to suffer mental illnesses like depression, stress, worry, fear, and phobias. We can become critical and judgmental of others and blame others instead of taking responsibility for our lives.

When this chakra functions positively, we have good coordination and reflexes. We are clear in our thoughts and focused with our actions. We enjoy learning, and we take that knowledge and apply it to our everyday lives through action, ambition, and energy. We suffer very little from sickness and stress because the organs this chakra governs are healthy and flowing with a balanced amount of energy. We feel at peace with ourselves and function positively on an emotional and physical level.

A JOURNEY INTO THE SIXTH CHAKRA

To understand and use this information, let's take a personal journey into this sixth chakra—our third eye. Find a time to be quiet and sit comfortably, while you breathe, relax, and set the intention to witness and explore what happens when you focus on this chakra.

Physical Location: Center of the forehead above the eyes

Feel the area above and between your eyes on your forehead. This is your third eye. Let your mind focus on this part of your body.

Color: Indigo, midnight blue

Next picture the color indigo or midnight blue streaming into this chakra. You can visualize this as a spotlight or a liquid stream of indigo entering your body at the site of this chakra. Take your time. Feel the vibration of this color. What do you sense? What are you experiencing in this part of your body? Notice sensations, images, or anything that is happening to you in this moment. Do not judge what happens. Just be an observer.

Element: Presence, inner sound

Everyone has a presence, a sense of how we are in the world. Some feel a strong sense of presence; others hardly seem to be here at all. How do you perceive your presence? When you allow yourself to get very quiet, you will "hear" an inner sound. Sometimes it seems like a hum; other times it can be loud, like a buzzing. Let yourself get quiet, and listen for your inner sound.

Area of the Body Governed: Brain, neurological system, eyes, ears, nose, pituitary and pineal glands

Now focus on your head. Let your awareness move from your eyes, ears, and nose to inside your head—your brain, your pituitary gland, and your pineal gland. Sense how this part of your body connects with the rest of you.

Qualities of the Brow Chakra: Center of psychic power and intuition, imagination, source of insight, spiritual energy, knowingness, wisdom, perception, experiences cosmic consciousness, telepathy, astral travel

Set your intention to focus on the qualities that this chakra represents. How can you enjoy these qualities in a balanced way? Do you give yourself time to imagine, to expand your perceptions to how you experience your intuition? Let that happen now.

Body System or Organ: Pituitary gland

Next bring your awareness to your pituitary gland inside your brain. Picture this part of your body as healthy, vital, and alive. Combine this awareness with the sensation/vibration of the color indigo or midnight blue. Notice any sensations in this part of your body. Is this color in this part of your body comfortable or not? How can you experience the subtle workings of this powerful gland in your body?

Physical Problems If Out of Balance: Mental illnesses such as depression, stress and worry, suffering from fears and phobias

Do you have any of the above dis-eases/conditions? How strong is your body? This is a time to focus on your health and the vitality that you want to experience. Picture yourself full of energy, enthusiasm, and enjoyment. Do not judge your condition; let it teach you the lessons it has to improve your focus on your healing process.

Information Stored in the Brow Chakra: Seeing a clear picture (symbolic or literal), wisdom, intuition, mental faculties and intellect

When you are quiet, inside and out, there are times when you can see a picture—some call it a vision. What can you do to stimulate this part of your brain? How can you expand your wisdom?

Mental/Emotional Issues: Fear of truth, discipline, judgment, evaluation, emotional intelligence, concept of reality, and confusion

Judgment, confusion, and fear are emotions that can take over our lives. Fortunately, we do not have to give way to the negative side of our thoughts. Discerning between confusion and reality/truth and finding our emotional intelligence are difficult tasks. Be gentle with yourself in exploring these areas of your thinking and being. Be open to healing your mental and emotional issues.

Underactive Brow Issues: Doubting, envious of others' talents, forgetful, superstitious

When the energy in this chakra is **underactive** or blocked, there can be issues to deal with. Do you have problems with the qualities that are associated with this chakra being out of balance? This is a wonderful time to see how you can free yourself of qualities you no longer need or want.

Overactive Brow Issues: Worrying, fearful, oversensitive, impatient, belittling, egomaniac, authoritarian, ungracious, bitter

When the energy in this chakra is **overactive** or blocked, there can be issues to deal with. Do you have problems with the qualities that are associated with this chakra being out of balance? This is a wonderful time to be honest with yourself and see how you can free yourself of qualities you no longer need or want.

Spiritual Lesson: Understanding, reality checks, detachment, and open mind

How can you use the spiritual lessons of this chakra? How do they apply to you? What do you do to understand yourself, others, life? What processes do you use to make a reality check? Do you have the ability to detach in situations where you feel strongly about something? Can you let your mind stay open to hear both sides of an issue? Or do you make up your mind ahead of time and stick to a position with stubbornness? Let yourself ponder these questions and observe how you are with the answers. Again, be a witness to the process.

Chakra Truth: Search for the truth and trust. Never give up on your search for the difference between truth and fallacy. Trust the truth in Divine guidance.

Truth and trust—how do we let ourselves experience the difference between truth and illusion, between fear and trust? You have chosen to become a healer. That means you will be one who continually searches for the truth, discarding illusions (fear = false evidence appearing real).

Let yourself make this journey with the conviction of your faith. Know that you will be supported along your journey. You are entering a world where "believing is seeing" and leaving behind the world of "seeing is believing."

As this center also includes the organs of sight, ponder how you see the world. How do you face each day—with gratitude or with grumpiness? Are you experiencing fears or false impressions from your life? Begin now to let go of your fears. Send love and light to everything you fear. Healing is a choice that only you make possible.

Healing is knowing that the integration of your body, mind, and spirit will have a positive impact on your state of health. Healing is accepting self-responsibility and taking charge of your own life. Healing is loving and accepting your whole self.

NOTES FOR THE SIXTH CHAKRA

Acknowledge and identify any negative attitudes, beliefs, or perceptions.

Are you feeling judgmental about yourself and others?

Is your mind filled with generating illusions, false truth, or fears?

Trust in your healing.

The Seventh Chakra, Crown (Sahasrara)

The crown chakra is situated at the top of the head. This chakra governs part of the spinal cord, the brain stem, the pain center, and the nervous system.

On a spiritual level, the crown chakra, whose Sanskrit name is "Sahasrara," meaning thousandfold, is our connection to healing and life force energy. With a properly functioning crown chakra, we find fulfillment, self-realization, enlightenment, and Divine wisdom. We use the seventh chakra as a tool to communicate with our spiritual guides and angels. Through this crown chakra the life force energy gets dispersed from the universe into the lower six chakras to promote healing within us. This is the chakra that can create miracles. If we believe and have hope, working with this chakra can bring about true healing on all levels. When the crown is open, we become healthy physically, emotionally, mentally, and spiritually. An unblocked crown chakra frees us from depression, apathy, fear, and confusion. This chakra brings us to a higher awareness and a clear state of consciousness.

This chakra is the connection that we have to the Divine's unconditional love and beauty. When we believe, we are open to learning and to life's experiences that challenge us to grow and evolve into an aware individual. When we open ourselves to unconditional love, we allow ourselves to accept all beings. We are free from judgment toward others and their beliefs. We embrace the concept that "All Is One."

When the crown is enlightened, we radiate love and peace to all those around us. At the crown, we are able to free our limitations from our human brain and immerse ourselves in the Divine truth.

The crown chakra is associated with the colors white and violet to purple. These colors vibrate at an energy level that opens up our imagination and intuition. This center is connected to our higher mind/higher self. Our higher mind/higher self is the part of us that knows all the answers. It is the center of knowing without thought or reason. Here, the physical, emotional, intellectual, and spiritual integrates into the whole.

When our crown chakra opens, we rededicate our lives to whatever we feel is most important—loving others, maintaining peace, teaching, healing, and fostering our spiritual growth and the spiritual growth of others. It is here that we surrender to that which is so much greater than we are, but of which we are a part.

A JOURNEY INTO THE SEVENTH CHAKRA

To understand and use this information, let's take a personal journey into this seventh chakra—our crown chakra. Find a time to be quiet and sit comfortably, while you breathe, relax, and set the intention to witness and explore what happens when you focus on this chakra.

Physical Location: Top of the head

Close your eyes and gently breathe while focusing on the top of your head—and beyond. Let your mind hone in on this part of your body, then expand beyond.

Color: Violet/white

Next picture the color violet or white streaming into this chakra. You can visualize this as a spotlight or a liquid stream of violet entering your body at the site of this chakra. Take your time. Sense the vibration of this color. What do you feel? What are you experiencing in this part of your body? Notice sensations, images, or anything that is happening to you in this moment. Do not judge what happens. Just be an observer.

Element: Ether, the heavens

This chakra takes us beyond our physical bodies and into the realms above us, into the heavens, our ethereal body.

Area of the Body Governed: Top center of the head, the brain midline above the ears, and the entire nervous system

Now focus on the top of your head and how your entire nervous system starts here and travels throughout your body. Be a mind explorer and take a journey through your nervous system. Like a camera that could travel inside your body, let your thoughts follow the path of your nerves.

Qualities of the Crown Chakra: Divine awareness, our oneness with all, spiritual, faithful, peaceful, joyful, grateful, love of beauty, total access to the unconscious

Set your intention to focus on the qualities that this chakra represents. How can you enjoy these qualities in a balanced way? How can you experience oneness with all?

Body System or Organ: Pineal gland

Next bring your awareness to your pineal gland deep in your brain at the top of your brain stem. Picture this part of your body as healthy, vital, and alive. Combine this awareness with the sensation/vibration of the color violet or white. Notice any sensations in this part of your body. Is the color violet in this part of your body comfortable or not? Know that the pineal gland is functioning properly.

Physical Problems If Out of Balance: Sense of frustration, depressed, frequent migraines, full of despair, egotistical, destructive, sometimes distant

Do you have any of the above dis-eases/conditions? How strong is your body? This is a time to focus on your health and the vitality that you want to experience. Picture yourself full of energy, enthusiasm, and enjoyment. Do not judge your condition; let it teach you the lessons it has to improve your focus on your healing process.

Information Stored in the Crown Chakra: Concept of the whole

How connected do you feel to the whole—the whole of humanity, the whole of the world, the whole of the universe? How does that connection present itself to you? This is a time to expand your thinking—outside the body.

Mental/Emotional Issues: Discovery of the Divine, lack of purpose, loss of meaning or identity, trust, selflessness, humanitarianism, ability to see the bigger picture in the life stream, devotion, inspiration, values, and ethics

Now search deep inside yourself. Take your time. Be honest and let the healing process take place. Do you know what your purpose and meaning in life are? Trust in your ability to see the bigger picture in life. Feel the inspiration and devotion from the Divine.

Underactive Crown Issues: Lacking tenderness, shame, self-denial and negative self-image, cannot make decisions, lack of memory, no fun or joy in life

When the energy in this chakra is **underactive** or blocked, there can be issues to deal with. Do you have problems with the qualities that are associated with this chakra being out of balance? This is a wonderful time to be honest with yourself and see how you can free yourself of qualities you no longer need or want.

Overactive Crown Issues: Needing to feel popular and indispensable, intense imagination

When the energy in this chakra is **overactive** or blocked, there can be issues to deal with. Do you have problems with the qualities that are associated with this chakra being out of balance? This is a wonderful time to be honest with yourself and see how you can free yourself of qualities you no longer need or want.

Spiritual Lesson: Spirituality and living in the now, to be one with the Source

How can you use the spiritual lessons of this chakra? How do they apply to you? Do you live and dwell in the past? Do you live for tomorrow? Or do you live in the present moment? Search inside and, if you want to know an answer to something, direct your attention with the oneness of the Divine. Everything exists within you.

Chakra Truth: Live in the present moment.

Achieve your own special relationship with the Divine. Remove any illusions or fears and any false impressions from your life. Let go of living in the past. Do not wait for the future to happen, because we do not know what tomorrow brings. Live in the presence of the Divine and in the *now*.

NOTES FOR THE SEVENTH CHAKRA

Acknowledge and identify what has happened in your life today.

Are you living in the moment or in the past or future?

Do you bless every day with gratitude and love?

Trust in your healing.

What Have You Learned about Yourself Up to This Point?

Take out a piece of paper or open your computer and write down at least five changes you have noticed since you started reading about the chakras and exploring what significance they have on your life.

Now that you have personally connected with each of your energy centers and have a better understanding of the chakras, see if you can answer the following questions.

- Explain the concept of the existence of universal and human energy.

- List the seven energy centers (chakras) in the body and their locations.

- Identify the function of each of the chakras.

- Explain how/why each chakra becomes blocked.

- List specific illnesses that can be caused by blocked energy centers in the body.

- Define how to resolve blockages of energy in the chakras.

Here are some questions to ask yourself to help you work out what the underlying cause of an illness might be:

- Why do some people get sick and others don't?

- How is it that some people can eat a healthful diet and exercise, yet still develop chronic illnesses?

- Why is it that some people are so comfortable playing the "sick and victim" role?

- What should I do to truly love and accept myself?

- What is it that I need to be made aware of to learn about myself and my body?

- What changes in my life do I need to make in order to become healthy and whole again?

- What is it that I may be ignoring in my life that needs changing?

- My body needs something from me and has developed this sickness. What does it need?

- What is it that I am ignoring in my life?

Remember this is all a process of growth and healing and the ability to live a wonderful healthy life. When we have our health, we are very wealthy.

CHAPTER 3

Auras and Protecting Your Energy

We are all susceptible to our own and each other's energies, and one of the most common reasons people become ill is because of negative thoughts, words, or behaviors of their own or those directed at them by another person. Anyone can pick up negativity from another person. Situations we encounter can leave us feeling exhausted and/or ill with a headache, nausea, backache, chest or neck pain, or other symptoms, whether spiritual, physical, or emotional.

Others may feel as if their body is suddenly sluggish or weighed down. The body's energy field (aura) is picking up energy field disturbances (negative energy) from other individuals, causing the body mental, physical, emotional, or spiritual problems or discomfort.

Let's say, for example, you are going to visiting a friend. From the very moment you walk through the door of her home, your friend does nothing but complain and is extremely negative. Every word from her mouth is a complaint. You sympathize and listen to every word, not realizing that their negative energies are affecting you by attaching to your aura.

Keep in mind that if this person has been negative for most of her life or has lived in a toxic environment at the same location for a long time, negative energy lingers all around the home. Every nook and cranny, in every room, has an energetic residue left behind from thoughts and/or negative influences and vibrations.

When you finally get the courage to leave the house and get into your car, you realize that your body feels drained and fatigued from all the negativity, complaining, and toxicity in that home. What do you think has happened here? Your friend's negative energies and the toxicity in the home have attached to your aura. The negative energies may cause you to have a headache, backache, and feel exhausted, and now you are becoming slightly irritable. Does this sound familiar?

This is an example of how your immune system and energy field can be weakened when you have been surrounded by negative energy. At the end of the day, you may find you have been with other people at work or socially and accumulated a lot of energetic debris; in other words, you've accumulated "energy static cling." These energies have become attached to your own energy field and leave you feeling drained. The more aware you become of this, the more you can prevent it from happening.

However, not all energy intrusion comes from other people. Our own fear, negative thoughts, expressions, feelings, and actions can cause us to experience energy uneasiness too. Negative thought patterns attract feelings of anxiety, fear, and constant worry and panic that can create problems. When you find yourself experiencing road rage, a temper tantrum, getting into an argument with someone, or just being impatient in the grocery store line, take a step back and ask yourself, "Why am I allowing this negative energy to affect my emotions?" It is very important to become aware of your actions and the energies that are producing your negative emotions.

Ask yourself this question: Is this negativity I am experiencing coming from myself or outside influences or both? If this is a symptom of energy contamination, you can take measures to prevent it. Become aware of the answer and of your feelings and begin to take charge; then change the situation or outcome. Remember, positive brings positive, negative brings negative.

Whether we realize it or not, we are all frequently exposed to foreign energy fields. On a daily basis we come into contact with energy from other people that we have little or no control over. Our energy fields are like magnets, and as a result, we can often take on energy that is not ours. Some of this energy can be positive and healthy, but some can be negative and not so good for us and adversely affect our well-being. We can walk out of our own house feeling fine, but come home feeling tired or drained. We can feel "off" or "ill" for reasons we cannot understand or explain. More often than not, it is because we have been energetically affected by our contact with other people, places, or things.

What Is an Aura?

Another word for energy field is aura. The dictionary defines *aura* in many ways, one of which is, "a distinctive atmosphere surrounding a person, such as an aura of sanctity." Simply put, your aura is a multilayered energy field that surrounds your body and intermingles with the atmosphere of the earth and all other forms of life. Your aura protects you by filtering out some of the energies you encounter and drawing in others that you may need. Our aura is like the wind, felt but not readily seen. About seventy-five years ago, a man named Kirlian happened onto a photographic technique that enables us to see these auras. With Kirlian photography, scientists have been able to study and observe the auras of plants, human hands, even the entire human body. What we can see is that auras have specific characteristics—different colors, textures, shapes, and densities.

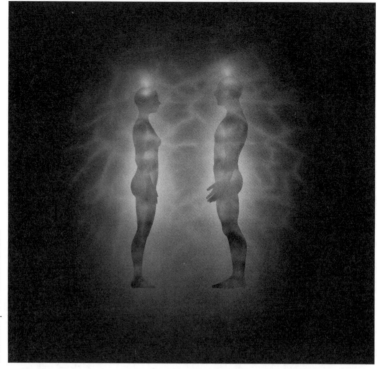

Our aura permeates and energizes us physically, emotionally, mentally, and spiritually. It reveals our state of health, our "ease" or "dis-ease." When we feel healthy, happy, contented, and energetic, the aura tends to be large and bright and can fill an entire room. When we are sick, sad, and depressed or constantly complaining, our aura tends to be small and dark, forming an energetic shell around the body that can isolate us from other people.

The aura has many electromagnetic energy patterns that expand beyond our physical body. Everything living and nonliving has a unique energy field that constantly vibrates at its own frequency. Our body is unable to support life without its aura. Just think of what would happen to the earth without the atmosphere. Our auras are our energetic atmospheres.

Wherever we come into contact with other people, their thoughts and their energies intermingle with ours and with all life-forms. We are all a part of the universe and the energy within it. Our aura is constantly connecting with other energy fields. When this happens, a wave is sent through it, the same as when a pebble falls into water. The vibrations reach around our aura and into our physical system. The brain notices the sensation and then interprets the experience for us. As an example: When we are in a room with many people and one person begins an argument with another, our energy field meets that of the arguing individuals, and a wave of uneasiness is created around our aura where the energies meet. This feeling ripples through our body and our consciousness. Our hair literally stands on end because of this arguing, and our brain interprets this sensation as fear and we begin to feel very uncomfortable.

This is what is known as energy intrusion within the aura, causing our physical body to experience a feeling of stress. A contrary example: If we are on vacation and decide to relax by a beautiful blue/green ocean, the beauty is not only seen through our eyes but felt by our whole body. As in the previous example, the wave is felt in the physical body, but this time we experience relaxation and peacefulness. It is the same energy intrusion, but one is negative and one is positive.

Your aura can become weakened due to poor health, lack of exercise, stress, anxiety, overwork, and negative behavior. If you don't take good care of yourself, don't eat wholesome food or get sufficient fresh air or rest, your aura will weaken—and that in turn makes you more susceptible to other people's negativity. If you watch negative or violent television shows, if you tend to overthink or constantly worry, assume the worst, gossip, lie, or grip too tightly to the past or future—all these things can be both signs of a weakened aura and cause for further weakening.

Negative habits such as alcohol, drug, and/or tobacco consumption also contribute to feeling tired, drained, or sick. Chronic pain, inability to concentrate, memory loss, insomnia, and not being able to complete what you start—these are all part of the condition of a weakened aura. A weakened aura can sabotage us with negative thoughts and behaviors that create a toxic environment.

By taking steps to strengthen your aura, you become more vibrant and healthy, more respectful of your body, and less likely to be influenced and impinged upon by external situations. A strong aura can usually repel or stop outside negativity, preventing imbalances on all levels. A person with a strong aura thinks positively and usually takes responsibility for what they create in life and participates in a personal healing process. Strengthening or protecting your aura is well within your control!

One way to protect your aura is through what's called "energy protection." Energy protection is a defensive screen around the aura that safeguards our inner and outer space. This invisible barrier protects us from other people's thoughts and negative energies, whether they are intentional or unintentional.

It all starts with awareness. By being observant of sensations occurring from outside our body, such as the sounds that we hear and feelings of the space we occupy and the people around us, we can become aware of the need for protection. Personal observations that indicate the need of protection include feelings of annoyance, impatience, anger, and anxiousness.

There are several good ways to protect your aura. Through the years, I have worked with many individuals, including physicians, who have asked me to do spiritual healings on them or to teach them Gentle Energy Touch. I have encountered various types of energy field disturbances and have personally used the different techniques that worked for me. These are basic techniques anyone can use. You will know which techniques are correct as the ones that promote a feeling of comfort. I have always found that my inner guidance has been my best pilot.

Intention and knowledge are the most important factors for effective protection. Knowledge is power. The more knowledge-able and understanding we are, the less likely we are to run into problems. We become strong and unafraid, knowing that once we use common sense and are aware of our surroundings, we have the ability to recognize the negative influences around us.

The next step is learning to safeguard ourselves from being affected by individuals who may be unfavorable or troublesome to us physically and/or spiritually. Knowledge and awareness enable us to strengthen our energies, enhance our abilities, and prevent problems from developing. Energy follows thought. Where we put our thoughts is where our energy goes. Our thoughts manifest what we experience.

If a person believes they will catch the flu every winter, as winter approaches the mind tells the body, "You will catch the flu this winter." Guess what? That individual gets the flu and is the first one to say, "See, I told you I would get the flu." This thought and intention leaves the individual open and susceptible to catching the flu. We create our own self-fulfilling predictions in most instances.

Practically speaking, we need to respect our body, get enough sleep, eat healthily, drink plenty of water, do not skip meals, and get enough physical exercise. Physical and energetic health is all connected. When we are physically and mentally exhausted, combined with a feeling of extreme nervousness, our aura can be more easily affected by people and/or changes around us.

Most important, we need to keep our surroundings free from negativity. The key is to stop making excuses and become aware of our needs. Maybe it's time to begin setting boundaries and taking care of yourself. Take that well-deserved day off from work; sleep that extra hour on the weekend; begin to exercise and eat healthily and take a few minutes just to sit still and breathe and relax. Stop and/or cut down on drinking alcohol, smoking, or using drugs, and just don't answer the phone if you need quiet time. When we do this, we begin to take control of our life and help ourselves accomplish what needs to be done physically, emotionally, mentally, and spiritually. Only we have the ability to choose to do so.

In order to do energy protection effectively, it is important to stay positive and eliminate preconceptions. First, gently breathe and affirm yourself, knowing, trusting, and feeling that Divine energy is always there to protect you. Remember and reaffirm that you are in control of the choices you make at all times. By doing this you show that you do not allow unwholesome energies into your aura. Saying positive affirmations aloud or silently, such as "I am open to the best and closed to the undesirable," will work to protect your aura from unwanted energies.

The power of the imagination is beyond measure. Whatever we can imagine and believe in, we can bring into being. To believe in ourselves is one of the strongest protections we have. Knowing at the deepest level of our being that nothing can touch us is one of the perfect protections. The other perfect protection is sending out love.

Exercises for Sensing Energy

Let's look at how to recognize what your own aura feels like and how to sense the flow of energy around your body.

You are composed of energy that flows within and around you. How do you know this when you cannot see it? How do you know that energy healing is beneficial for treating many illnesses when you cannot physically observe the energy you are working with?

In fact, many of us have experienced feeling other people's energy but have probably never realized it. Have you ever had the sensation that someone was watching you? Have you ever felt someone come into a room from behind you? When you enter a room full of people, have you been drawn to sit next to or avoid a certain person? Of course you have. What you were feeling and sensing was the other person's energy. Some people's auras extend as far as the outstretched arms and the full length of the body. Others who are spiritual and evolved can extend up to sixty-five feet or more beyond the physical body. Your own aura picks up on the energies from the other person.

The following are some exercises you can do that will allow you to actually sense the energy. The first step is to relax, take some deep breaths, and ground yourself in Mother Earth. This will help you focus and concentrate on feeling the energy. (See page 174 for grounding technique.)

EXERCISE #1

This exercise is done with the intention of activating the energy in the hands. Start by shaking both hands for fifteen seconds. Then place the thumb of one hand in the palm of the other hand approximately one and a half inches in from the base of the thumb and above the wrist. Press for ten seconds. Repeat the same procedure on the other hand.

Hold your hands open in front of you, about twelve inches apart, with the palms facing each other. Concentrate on the feelings in your palms; then slowly move your hands toward each other. If you do not feel anything, move your hands a little farther apart. Again, slowly move your hands toward each other. You may have to do this several times, each time keeping your hands farther apart then before.

When you start to feel a little resistance between your hands or a little tingling sensation, you are now sensing the energy surrounding your body. Continue this exercise by moving your hands farther apart, then checking for any sensations in your palms as you bring them together. Notice how far away your hands can be and still touch your energy!

When you first do this, you may experience only a slight sensation—resistance, heat, tingling—or nothing at all. Be persistent; keep trying! Eventually you will feel it. Once your hands reach a point where you feel the energy between them, keep your hands at that distance and begin to move your hands around the energy field in a circle. It will feel as if you have a ball or a sphere in your hands!

You have now had your first experience working with energy!

EXERCISE #2

This is done with two people, sitting or standing and facing each other. Each raises their hands in front keeping them approximately six to twelve inches from the other person's hands. Feel for any pressure, tingling, or heat from the other person's hands.

If you don't feel anything, move your hands closer together or farther apart from each other until you do. When you feel sensations in your palms, continue to back up from each other and see how far apart you can get and still feel the energy.

You will be amazed at how far apart you can be and how far from your body your energy extends!

EXERCISE #3

This exercise requires three people. The first person sits in a chair, the second person stands behind the chair, and the third person kneels in front of the individual who is seated and places a hand on each of that person's knees.

To begin, the individual standing behind the chair puts their hands on the shoulders of the person who is seated, then closes their eyes. The stander then begins to think about sending energy through the seated individual into that person's knees. You might visualize this as a continuous stream or pulsing waves of energy.

The kneeler now closes their eyes and concentrates on their own hands, feeling for any sensations such as heat or tingling. As the stander strengthens thought intensity to increase the energy flowing through the seated person, the kneeler should also feel an increase in sensation.

All three individuals should take turns at the different positions so each may experience the exercise.

Congratulations! You have now experienced something that most people have never felt—an awareness of the energy that we all have in and around our bodies. This energy is what you will work with while using Gentle Energy Touch to help yourself heal.

Protecting Your Aura

As with anything new, it takes time and patience to put these spiritual techniques into practice. Do not procrastinate! Always stay grounded, centered, balanced, and calm. Gently breathe and become aware of where you are and, most important, . . . *do it!* Remember that being strong is not only about physical power. Toughness is connected with the mind, and when you are strong, you possess adequate mental strength.

Having a strong and healthy mind can help you a lot in achieving your dreams and goals. When you stay positive, you improve the strength of your mind, and you will possess valuable qualities like determination, persistence, passion, tranquility, dedication, and patience, just to name a few. A strong mind can cope with a weak body, while even a strong body is no use if you have a weak mind. Healing is recognizing that you have the ability to be able to command your thoughts and do anything you set your mind to do. Remember that your aura is simply an extension of you. When strong, it acts as a protective shield. When fragile or damaged, it can leave you drained, unwell, and feeling disconnected from yourself.

As you practice the following protection techniques, take the time to breathe and relax for a few moments and to visualize your aura surrounded with white and golden protective light, encasing you from your head down to and under your feet.

Remember: The *intention* of protecting your energy field is what protects you. There must never be any fear or doubt. When you create a protective shield, it is important to have a firm conviction that it is there, it protects you, and it cannot be penetrated by unwanted energies. If at any time you show signs of fear, doubt, or anger, your protective shield weakens and can be penetrable. Just a note: you can apply a protective shield around other people such as a child, for instance, who may be bullied at school. You can put protective light around your home, car, and any other items you wish to protect. Everything has an aura, and mostly everything needs some form of energy protection.

When using any form of protection, always send negative energy down to Mother Earth with love and light and healing; we want the negative energy to heal. (More on this below.) Trust your inner guidance and follow your intuition.

NINE EXCELLENT METHODS OF
ENERGY PROTECTION

1. Close Your Aura

One of the easiest ways to protect yourself is to make your aura dense and compact. This can be done instantly and means the aura is more difficult to penetrate. Closing your aura is a conscious form of energy protection.

To keep your aura completely dense and close to your body, cross your legs and put your hands together on your lap or the lower abdominal area. There is no need to visualize anything, just use your intention to close the aura. This technique is effective when you are around people at a business meeting, a party, in an airport, etc. It prevents individuals from draining your energy. When you have moved away into a safe space and are no longer subject to energy depletion, set the intention to open your aura to receive love and light and for the same to go out to others.

2. Become Nonreactive

When someone gets very angry with you and you do not show a reaction to that negative emotion, have you noticed that they get angrier? The anger directed toward you bounces back to the individual, creating more of an imbalance around that person's energy field. What you can do to protect your own energy in such situations is to stay calm and remain detached. Then you will not be energetically affected by their anger. You must be the one to think clearly and respond without attachment to the emotional outburst as long as you are not in danger. Attempt to get the angered individual out of the angry mindset. Sometimes just saying "I am sorry" or "how can I help you?" or simply listening without interrupting can decrease the anger directed at you.

When you react to someone's anger, you become vulnerable to the negative thought forms that person is throwing out, allowing the negativity to attach to your aura. Remaining in a neutral and positive state is extremely important. Visualize, imagine, and silently chant "peace," "shanti," "shalom," "love and light," or "peace is with you." Concentrate on your heart. Bless the person with love and the intention that this negative energy becomes calm, loving, peaceful, and understanding. You will also feel better about doing this because your own energy will not be depleted. I know it is sometimes difficult to focus on love when someone is screaming at you, but remain calm and you will see the effect on you reduced.

3. Protect Yourself through Loving

Love is a positive and creative force that repels negativity. It empowers you because the strength of love will block any attacking energy and push it away. Negative energy cannot attach itself when you do not welcome unhealthy attitudes or negative vibrations. Always feel and think loving thoughts. I always say to myself "love and light" to those I come in contact with.

4. Send Negative Energy into the Earth

When you feel negative energies around you, simply close your eyes, breathe, and with every exhale ask the energy to leave while you visualize sending it down into Mother Earth with love and light and healing. Continue sending and visualizing until you feel your aura is clear and lighter energetically. Remember positive intention creates positive reality.

When Mother Earth receives this unwanted energy, she recycles it into positive energy, sending it back into the atmosphere. You may want to say a prayer when sending the negative energies to Mother Earth: "We are asking that Mother Earth blesses this energy with light, love, and power to be regenerated into positive energy." Just a note here, if you do not want to send the energies down to Mother Earth, visualize a bucket of fire and picture putting the energies in the bucket. Then ask God, the Divine, or to whomever you pray to remove the energies safely to be recycled into positive with love and light and healing.

5. Ask for Negative Energy to Be Removed

This simple technique is done with the intention of removing residual negative energies when handling, manufacturing, or distributing food, clothes, cosmetics, etc., that other people have handled. It is important to clear their energy from the products.

Place the palms of both hands over the food you are about to eat or beverage you are about to drink and ask for any unwanted energies to be removed. Ask for healing energies to be directed onto the food and water. Then eat and drink slowly, visualizing eating and drinking healing light. Do the same with cosmetics, clothes, and so on. Ask for the negative energies to be sent to Mother Earth with love and light and healing. Repeat this technique until you feel the items are clear of unwanted energies.

6. Cocoon Your Body

Imagine a protective (encircling) cocoon of white and golden light beginning from under your feet and going up around your legs, thighs, hips, waist, stomach, chest, heart, throat, face, and head and around the entire back of your body. Set the intention that any negative energy not penetrate this cocoon but that love spreads out to all people you come in contact with or any situation you encounter. You can cocoon yourself prior to going to work, traveling, having guests come in your home, or going out for a night of the town, etc.

7. Sweep It Away

I would like to mention that just as we need to clear our homes and workplace of clutter, our energetic fields must also be cleared of the old energy, thoughts, and emotions that do not serve us any longer. When we clear our aura and energy centers, it helps to restore and strengthen our connection to ourselves and to our

Divine inner wisdom. It is very important to rid our energy bodies of fear, pain, self-hatred, judging, or any other emotion that does not serve us well. When we do so, we are able to set ourselves free on a conscious level so our body, mind, and spirit has the ability to be free to grow.

The intention of sweeping is to remove all negative energies that may have attached to your aura. This technique is quick to use and works very well for those in contact with many people throughout the day.

Cup each hand, palms facing you, with fingers of each hand together and fingertips pointing toward each other about three inches apart. Begin about ten inches above your head and sweep your hands in a downward motion to your feet in front of your body. Visualize and set your intention to do the same sweeping motion down your back. Repeat the sweeping motion a few times until you feel the surrounding energy is lighter. Always sweep downward and never upward. Sweeping downward clears, but if you sweep upward, you can cause more energy congestion. Always send the negative energy to Mother Earth with love and light and healing to be recycled. Even though you are not touching the physical body while sweeping the aura, this motion heals and balances the aura and directly affects your physical health. The more you use this technique the more you will notice you are not being affected by other people's energies.

8. Vacuum It Away

The intention would be the same as in the sweeping practice example above. Instead of sweeping energy away, sit with your hands on your lap and visualize the nozzle of a vacuum cleaner beginning at the top of your head and moving slowly downward going around your body pulling out all the debris from your aura.

Make sure you go all the way down slowly to the bottom under your feet. Make sure you send the unwanted energies collected down to Mother Earth with love and light and healing. If you feel there is still unwanted energy, simply begin at the top of your head again and repeat.

This next technique is the one I use most. I saved it for last because not everyone feels comfortable invoking God, and I wanted to show you other options. But I feel the hand of God in what I do, and I always thank God for everything I receive. In my heart I know God is with me, I trust God is with me, and I feel God is with me! If prayers to God are not for you, I encourage you to make up your own words of prayer or affirmations that feel comfortable to you.

9. The White Light Bubble Technique

You can use this White Light Bubble Technique anywhere, at any time of the day, and as many times as you feel it is necessary. It is a simple and effective way to keep God close to you. It will not only protect you against negative thoughts or energies, it will constantly uplift your spirit.

Say the following White Light Prayer as you visualize a light sprinkle of the purest, cleansing rays of white and golden light pouring onto your head and covering your entire being, engulfing you in a bubble or a very close and tight outline. Visualize this light cleansing your body while creating an impenetrable barrier.

> *The Light of God Surrounds Me*
> *The Love of God Enfolds Me*
> *The Power of God Protects Me*
> *The Presence of God Watches Over Me*
> *Wherever I Am God Is, Amen*

—FROM JAMES DILLET FREEMAN

Here is another prayer of energy protection that you can say as you put yourself in a bubble of protective light: "All power is of God, what is not of God has no power to do anything to me."

Important! The bubble/outline technique keeps "out" negative energies, but it does not restrict the good energies of love from entering or leaving.

Try this technique a few times a day, beginning in the morning. While in the shower, visualize yourself under a shower or gentle waterfall of silver and golden cleansing light. Let this light pour over you, through you, and out into your surrounding aura, asking God to remove any negative energies that may have attached to your aura. Become aware of any heavy energy in your body and make a note of this observation to see if there is a pattern. Then send those energies down the drain into the earth with love and light so they may heal. If you feel heavy energies when you are out and about, just take a moment to go to a place where you are alone and visualize the same as above, sending the energies to Mother Earth with love and light so they may heal.

Surround yourself with white light when you're out and about. If you're sitting in a bus or train, on the way to work, or you're feeling stressed during the day, visualize the calming white and golden light pouring over you. Use the technique in the evening before retiring to bed, too.

It sounds too simple to be true, but it does work. Practicing this technique on a regular basis will improve the way you feel. (*Note:* This energy protection technique is spiritual in nature. The usage of God in these prayers does not represent any religion. Please use any prayer you feel comfortable with.)

For extra energy protection, use both or whatever prayer feels right for you. Either prayer can be handwritten on a piece of paper and put under the four corners of your mattress. The prayers will keep you safe while you sleep. If you need to clear the energies in your home or office, place the prayers in every corner of the room with the intention of clearing the energies. You can place the prayers in your desk drawers, your bag, your car—wherever you feel the need to clear. Always write them out by hand because there is power in your writing. Do not make copies, write every one on a separate piece of paper, and place them where needed . . . Yes it is a lot of writing, but you will feel the difference in energy in the areas you place them.

All the above techniques are suggestions. Let your all-knowing and inner guidance find the protection that feels right for you. Always come from pure unconditional love.

Our beautiful Mother Earth and the universe need empowered and loving human beings. Whether you clean streets, manage large companies, or are the president of the United States, your real contribution will come from the love, attitude, and positive energies you radiate.

Any kindness or love we show to one another will have a ripple effect throughout the world. When you are in line at the grocery store or in the mall or just walking down the street, the greatest energy work you can do is to smile at one another. Let's put a little love in our hearts and let it shine throughout the world.

Prana Energy and Healing

Another important concept to understand in energy healing is prana. Prana is the vital life force energy that exists in all living things. There are several sources of prana energy: solar, earth, air. Our body's primary source of life force is through the air we breathe—air prana. When we are outside in the sunlight, the body absorbs solar prana. Every time we take a breath, our body is absorbing air prana and when we walk on soil, sand, or any other natural surface, our body absorbs earth prana automatically and unconsciously. All living things require this energy to be nourished and sustain life. It is the activating energy of the universe, an electrical type of energy that gives life to the body and determines our state of health.

Prana is like a current that travels throughout our bodies, energizing each cell. Our body utilizes this "vital life force energy" to build, repair, and maintain itself. When prana is weak, depleted, or blocked, illness occurs. When prana energy is strong and flowing freely, we are healthy.

There are many factors that can cause prana energy to become weakened, such as contamination of the soil, air, and water. Chemically fertilized crops, for example, have a reduced nutritional value, longer shelf life, and higher resistance to both insects and disease. When the food we eat is grown in soil that is depleted of nutrients, our bodies don't get the nourishment they need to sustain life.

The same applies to the air we breathe and the water we drink. If the air is polluted with chemicals, what we breathe in adversely affects the cells and tissues in every part of our body. When the water is contaminated with chemicals, every sip we take compromises our health. Our body requires clean water to survive. As much as possible, try to eat organic foods and live someplace where the air and water are clean. This enables your vital life force energy level to remain high and your body to remain healthy.

Other factors can diminish or weaken our energy level as well. Our beliefs, emotions, past or present traumatic memories, our attitude, what we say, how we react to situations, where we work and live all influence the state of our health. When you are considering what might be causing your own life force energy to become depleted, look in all the following areas.

1. **Emotional.** Worrying or being fearful that you will not have enough money to pay your bills, getting laid off from your

job, getting a promotion (even though this usually is a good change, it can be stressful), arguing, having disagreements, conflicts, stress, anger, resentment, and depression (just to name a few) all cause energy depletion by actually draining your brain of vitality and focusing power.

2. **Physical.** Problems such as body ailments, illness, infection, pain, fractures or dislocations, or not getting enough sleep can weaken us. Also, pushing your body too hard such as working twelve hours a day and not having a good work/ life balance, hormonal factors such as puberty, premenstrual syndrome, postpartum fluctuations, and menopause (just to name a few) all cause stress on the body and deplete life force energy. Not getting enough exercise and sitting most of the day cause fatigue and energy depletion.

3. **Nutritional.** Deficiencies caused by food allergies, poor digestion, eating too much sugar and carbohydrates, not drinking enough water, drinking too much soda, eating too many processed foods, not having a balanced diet, insufficient vitamin and mineral intake, excessive caffeine, cigarette smoking, and alcohol or drug use all weaken our energy levels.

4. **Environmental.** Problems found in hot or cold climates such as heat exhaustion or hypothermia, toxins or poisons such as insecticides, car pollution, and smog all cause energy depletion in one's life. If you live and work in a negative environment, the prana you are breathing into your body is negative, causing ill effects. Also consider the impact of clutter, mess, and disorganization. A cluttered environment tends to clutter our minds. Prana energy is the very essence that keeps us alive. Strong, free-flowing prana is vital for our good health. The quality of everything we do, including breathing, sensing, eating, moving, feeling, thinking,

playing, working, communicating, loving, etc., all depends on how we manage our lives and our energy. Living in a positive environment allows us to breathe in positive prana, promoting good health. The importance of prana healing cannot be emphasized enough. It is essential in helping us maintain a healthy body, mind, and spirit.

We are all energy transmitters connected with the whole of the universe: **All is One.**

There are two main techniques used in prana healing: scanning and sweeping/clearing. Unlike traditional Reiki or energy healing, prana healing does not require touching the body. I'll be teaching you how to do scanning and sweeping in chapter 6.

CHAPTER 4

Expect a Cleansing Period

As you begin to practice the self-healing treatments, you may experience a "cleansing" period. The mind and body are being stimulated to release toxins, along with feelings and emotions that are no longer needed. This cleansing period shows that the healing process is active and that toxins are leaving the body.

It manifests differently for each person. Some may experience sweating, headaches, minor illnesses such as a cold or influenza, the need to sleep more, the need to drink more fluids, mood changes, unusual dreams, or other emotional and physical changes. The opposite is also possible, and some individuals may feel totally renewed and revitalized. Some may notice that certain physical symptoms may disappear immediately or may take a few days to begin feeling better. Keep a journal during this process to record changes that do occur to see your progress.

Each treatment may activate a different form of cleansing as the energy centers adjust to the higher vibration. When cleansing of the emotional body occurs, deeply held feelings such as anger, frustration, grief, fear, and sadness might surface for no obvious reason. These emotions may have been repressed or suppressed from earlier in this lifetime or even from past-life experiences. They are being released at the cellular level of the body and mind. Do not judge these feelings. Experience them as they come up and then let them go. If this should occur for you, it is important to understand what is happening and to support it until its conclusion. Some changes may be minor, while others may alter your whole perspective and how you approach life, opening you to a new outlook.

Issues long forgotten may emerge and require addressing so you can go on with life in a healthy way. Usually, a period of adjustment is necessary to become accustomed to a healthier state of being. More rest or quiet time may be required to contemplate the changes that need to be made. Look at this as a period of cleansing. Do not be afraid; rather, work with it to put your life back on track for a fresh new beginning.

Everything has its own vibration rate. Negative thoughts and emotional patterns (negative energy) have a lower vibratory rate than the waves of energy we create when thinking positive thoughts. When you do a healing treatment, the sudden increase in the flow of positive energy will loosen the negative energy that has been blocked within your body making you ill. This will allow old blockages of stored up negative emotions and memories to be released, as this is necessary for further growth.

Although this change maybe sudden, it takes time for the adjustments to become effective. It takes approximately three days for the energy to move through each of the seven major chakras (crown, third eye, throat, heart, solar plexus, sacral, root). The opening of the energy channel occurs in the upper half of the body from the crown down to the heart chakra (channeling heavenly energy) and from the energy centers in the lower part of the body from the legs up through the root, also ending at the heart chakra (channeling earth energy).

Some people feel as if life becomes more difficult when they begin doing self-healing sessions. The truth is that the healing sessions are dredging up deep-seated energy blocks (emotional, physical, mental, or spiritual), and as individuals become more sensitive and aware of these issues, they must now work harder to focus and resolve them.

Dreams are another way of monitoring changes that may occur with your treatments. By continually reinforcing the suggestion to remember your dreams before retiring at night, you will eventually be able to recall them in better detail upon waking. Dreams are tools that help you tune in to the subconscious. Although they may seem senseless or unclear at times, with persistence, a pattern will begin to emerge that tells you about your inner self. It will usually disclose issues that need to be confronted. This is a good time to develop a habit of performing a healing treatment before going to sleep at night and when waking (after writing down your dreams) in the morning.

Continual healing sessions after the initial cleansing process will help foster spiritual growth and further refinement of energy flow. With spiritual cleansing, beliefs may be shaken and challenged. How you see the world operating, how you think relationships should be, what you feel about religion, what is important in your life, etc., could be called into question or need to be reexamined.

The insights, revelations, and new understanding that become clear in this process can become the building blocks of your newly forming and ever-changing spiritual foundation. A feeling of gratitude can increase and in turn create a greater level of abundance in many areas of your life. It can help you to manifest goals and desires, as well as heal troubling relationships. Where there is inconsistency and imbalance, energy healing can reinstate order and stability. No area is left untouched by the positive effects of self-healing.

When first beginning your treatments, make sure to give yourself a full self-healing treatment every day for twenty-one days (seven chakras taking three days each to cleanse).

Some cleansing periods may last as long as thirty days or more since the healing time can vary for each person. Do not skip a day; otherwise, the cleansing process and treatments will have to begin all over again at day one. Doing daily self-healing is an excellent way to shorten the cleansing time and negative effects that need to be cleared. This is a period for you to recognize and acknowledge what you are experiencing, then allow your feelings to heal by releasing the resentment and letting it go.

The twenty-one-day cleansing period is a positive process and necessary to fully clear and heal your energy centers. It is important to know that this is a temporary condition and part of a much-needed healing alignment. After your twenty-one-day cleansing period, take the time to continue doing healing on yourself at least three times a week. I do healing on myself every night. It keeps me clear, balanced, centered, and grounded, plus I continually let go of energies that do not serve me.

Be good to yourself and do not fear or stop the healing process that occurs. Let what needs to heal surface and be released. Receive it with open arms, knowing you've taken the first step in self-healing.

The following are suggestions that can help during the twenty-one-day cleansing period:

- Keep a daily journal of your feelings and experiences (including dreams).

- Be open to receiving the healing.

- Perform the self-healing techniques along with the chakra balancing and energy grounding techniques daily for twenty-one to thirty days. Remember to do your self-healing every day. If you miss a day, you will need to start at day one again, which just delays the cleansing process.

- Meditate or pray for at least ten to twenty minutes daily.

- Keep a peaceful, relaxed, and positive mind.

- Get adequate rest.

- Drink plenty of water to flush out any toxins that need to be released from the body.

- Eat healthful, nourishing foods and consider a brief water or juice fast, but only if you have experienced fasting in the past.

- Reduce or eliminate intake of alcohol, coffee, tea, chocolate, sweets, sugar, or other refined foods.

- Share your feelings or experiences with a supportive and trusted person.

- Do all things in moderation.

- Avoid confrontational or stressful situations.

- Reduce time watching television unless the programs are positive and inspirational.

- Be aware of your actions and surroundings.

- Be conscious of your own feelings and attitude.

- Understand and appreciate the feeling of calmness.

- Be open to loving yourself, the people around you, and your surroundings.

It is very important to recognize and understand the healing process and its implications. If anything negative surfaces as a result of the treatments, it is the body's way of releasing what it does not need anymore. This is necessary and should be seen as something good. This is a learning and growth process. Trust and listen to your inner guidance. Your new beginning has just gotten underway!

Part II

THE GENTLE ENERGY
TOUCH SESSION

And now it is time to learn the form the GET session takes. Every session, whether you are working on yourself or a partner, has some essential elements. In my work, I have identified thirteen steps that make for a complete healing session.

Step 1: Prepare the space.

Step 2: Set the intention for treatment.

Step 3: Asking for healing energy.

Step 4: Sweep and clear the aura.

Step 5: Begin the self-healing hand or partner table or chair positions.

Step 6: When treatment is finished, ask God to fill in all the voids with his healing light.

Step 7: Balance the chakras.

Step 8: Ground yourself (or your partner) to Mother Earth.

Step 9: Close the aura to keep the healing energies within the body.

Step 10: Give thanks for everything you have received.

Step 11: Disconnect from the energy or wash your hands with cold water.

Step 12: Drink a glass of water to help flush newly released toxins from the body.

Step 13: Receive feedback and have a conversation with your partner.

Now, let's begin.

CHAPTER 5

Setting the Stage for Healing

While you can learn how to practice Gentle Healing Touch on your own body, I suggest finding a partner to work with. Eventually you might even want to offer your services on a professional basis. But for now, let's assume you are concentrating on yourself or working with a friend/partner until you feel comfortable with the energy and the positions.

Prepare the Space

Let me start with a few pointers about preparing the space. It's so important for you to be in a serene setting, free from distractions, and that any person you are going to work with feels welcomed.

The appearance and atmosphere of the room you use should enhance the mood both for you and any other person receiving healing. Choose soft colors (if you can), keep the lights dim, and have some pleasant instrumental music playing at low volume. (You can find lots of good music for Reiki/healing through an Internet search, and I have put together some music resources in the back of the book.)

Using candles or fragranced oils with pleasant aromas can help create a healing atmosphere and have a calming effect on your partner, as long as they are not allergic to them. Always ask first. I usually use unscented white tea candles. They give the room a warm feeling and also help clear the energies and keep the room clear.

Also avoid wearing perfume and make sure to wash your hands with an unscented soap prior to doing a healing session in case the other person has sensitivities to certain odors.

Make sure your chair or table is at a height that is comfortable for you both. You may want to use a stool that can be moved around the table or chair easily without making noise if you are doing a session on a partner. There are many massage and/or Reiki tables available online. I have had an Earthlite table for the past twenty years. I believe the weight capacity is about 300 pounds. It is very durable. Both Amazon.com and Costco carry tables.

Keep the room at a comfortable temperature. Have towels or blankets easily accessible. Occasionally, a person's body temperature may drop when they become totally relaxed; you will then be prepared if you or your partner gets cold. Cover the table with a sheet and have pillows available to go under the head and/or knees.

Soft and positive conversation before and at the start of the treatment can put the person you are working with at ease. I do suggest being silent during the actual session to allow the receiver of the healing to experience any messages they are given. Some people may experience vivid colors or bright lights, may see certain images and memories (even past lives), and may experience emotional release. Just allow them to experience what needs healing and stay silent unless you are asked a question.

Keep noise levels to a minimum, and, if possible, shut off telephones, answering machines, beepers, and cell phones and close windows and doors to prevent possible distractions once the treatment begins.

Eat lightly two hours prior to a treatment and ask the person you will do the healing on to do so also.

Wear loose-fitting clothes for comfort when doing a self-healing or ask the person you will do the healing on to do so. Jewelry, tight belts, and shoes should be removed.

When doing GET for a woman, use a towel to cover the breasts, place her hands over her breasts, then place your hands over hers, or simply keep your hands one to two inches above the breasts (see hand positions in chapter 8). Prior to starting the healing, ask which she prefers.

Do not come in direct contact with another person's genital area. Simply keep your hands one to two inches above the area. Be respectful.

When properly prepared, both you and any partner experiencing the healing should find the treatment a rewarding experience.

Ask the receiver of the GET to close their eyes and relax. Remember it is all about helping the person to heal.

> *"Build a little fence of trust around today;*
> *Fill the space with loving work, and therein stay."*
> —MARY FRANCES BUTTS

Now that the space has been prepared, there are just two essential steps to take before you begin.

Set an Intention

I always recommend deciding on an intention or purpose for the treatment prior to doing Gentle Energy Touch. Consider for yourself or discuss with the partner you will be working on what they intend for the session. Observe how, in itself, coming up with an intention can set the healing process in motion. Just by thinking about this, you or your partner might discover an inner cause and/or solution to issues you've been holding deep inside, which would greatly increase the value of the Gentle Energy Touch and the help it brings. This often happens naturally, but stating an intention can speed up the process.

Be imaginative and don't set limits, but at the same time keep it simple. An example of a simple intent might be "to release tension and stress" or "to offer insight on a challenge or decision I am (she/he is) facing." Another example is to ask to "release any trauma from childhood or other times in my (her/his) life that serves no purpose now." When doing GET for a partner, it could be: "May I be a pure, energy-healing channel, and may this person receive everything he/she needs for his/her greatest good." When I do a session for someone else, I ask that person to say the intention to themselves for themselves. Also, once the intention is set, there is no need to constantly repeat it—just once is fine. Then ask your partner to just relax, close their eyes, listen to the music, and allow the healing to happen.

Writing down goals, hoped-for positive results, or any positive affirmations to heal problems is another way to make it easier for those issues to rise to the surface during the treatment, to be faced and resolved. Write down or ask your partner to write down some situations you or your partner may be looking to change. Put what you've written in an envelope to keep with you while doing GET. Have your partner hold the envelope while they receive treatment. During the treatment the body/mind/spirit will be very open to positive suggestions; therefore, it would be a good time to project affirmations to yourself or your partner both mentally and out loud.

Intention helps create reality by sending what we need out into the universe. We set in motion a process whereby what we intend will eventually come back to us. This is why it is important to be positive in our thoughts and have good intent in our actions. It is also just as important for the healer and receiver to be positive and know that the Gentle Energy Touch will help them in any manner they choose or release them from what it is necessary to be released from. Sometimes we may not know what it is that needs healing, but the energy we ask for is a very intelligent one and knows what we need. I also suggest that you and any friend you will be working on both give thanks for the life force energy you are about to receive.

The Gentle Energy Touch treatments are always successful. It is important to let this be clear in your mind and know and feel that it will. If you have doubts or reject its validity or really don't want it, but let it go on anyway, then you probably won't sense much at this time, although you may feel some small subtle changes in the future. So make your intentions positive and be open to the healing energy you are about to receive.

"Keep a grateful journal. Every night, list five things that you are grateful for. What it will begin to do is change your perspective of your day and your life."
—OPRAH WINFREY

Ask for Divine Healing Energy

Now it's time to ask for the assistance of Divine healing energy. Close your eyes and hold your hands (palms up) about twelve inches apart from each other. Ask God, the Divine, the Source, or the universe—whatever term feels comfortable to you—to ground you into Mother Earth and keep you balanced, centered, and coming from pure unconditional love.

Then say: "Dear God (the Divine, etc.), I ask for your healing energy for myself (your name or person's name) and to offer me (and them) the protection that I (and they) may need. I visualize myself (and them) in a bubble of protective white and golden light completely surrounding my (and their) aura. I call in from my (and their) higher self, archangels, angels, spirit guides, and loved ones all of the light to facilitate and assist me with your healing. God (the Divine, etc.), I also ask you to fill the room with your white protective light."

I like to add the following prayer:

The light of God surrounds me.
The love of God enfolds me.
The power of God protects me.
The presence of God watches over me.
Wherever I am God is.
Amen.

Then say: "Thank you, God (the Divine, etc.), for everything I am about to receive."

Also if you choose to do so, instead of saying this prayer at the beginning, you can say it at the end of the session, either for yourself or person you are working with.

Now begin visualizing the energy entering your crown chakra at the top of your head. Wait for that knowingness or sense that you have received the energy and feel it flowing through your hands. At this point you may notice tingling, heat, or heaviness sensations in your hands, as if they are magnetized. Once you feel the energy, begin with the first self-healing position (see p. 102).

Learn to trust your inner guidance and step out of your logical head for this to work.

Be patient: the energy does flow. As with anything new, it takes time and practice. The more often you do healing on yourself or a friend and become aware of the energy, the more intense the energy will be. Keep practicing, and know it is happening!

Here are other examples of prayers or techniques to use to ask for energy:

"I invoke the Master Spirits of Healing and ask that I be channeled with pure healing energy, without fear, with honor and love and provide me with the protection I may need."

"I align myself with the power of God's healing."

"Let me be a recipient for true loving healing."

"I invoke the angels of light, love, and healing. May I be receptive to the healing force and receive it with love."

"We are asking God/the Divine to shower his/its light, love, and healing on (name of person receiving the healing) for his/her highest good; and we are grateful for this."

"Dear God (the Divine, etc.), please offer healing, blessings, and life transformation as appropriate for this person." Please note that the words *as appropriate* are key. Never demand or force healing by saying you must get well or you must heal.

Please note: These are only a few suggestions for asking for energy. Say any prayer or technique you wish. The one that feels right for you is the one to choose. Please understand that I use the word God with no religion associated to it. One of my students calls in energy from the Holy Trinity and Jesus Christ. This helps make her Christian clients feel more comfortable. But it's entirely up to you how to ask for energy.

> *"What lies behind us and what lies before us are*
> *small matters to what lies within us."*
> —RALPH WALDO EMERSON

That's it! You are now ready to begin.

CHAPTER 6

Start with the Aura

Every Gentle Energy Touch session should begin with an aura scan. Scanning is a technique used to determine the areas where someone has energy congestion, an energetic blockage, an energetic deficiency, and/or leaking life force energy. This method helps you develop and use assessment skills and your own intuition to detect the areas on yourself or the other person that need healing energy. Also, scanning the aura removes any disturbing energies in the aura, and any person you are scanning will feel calmer and more prepared for treatment. After you have completed your Gentle Energy Touch session, you may scan the aura again, and this will help to settle or dispel excess or negative energies.

Scanning and asking for healing of someone's energy field is very beneficial, since illnesses originate here in the aura. When the aura is weak or is "leaking" life force energy, it can "expose" our bodies and make us vulnerable to negative influences that can affect us physically, mentally, emotionally, and/or spiritually, resulting in dis-ease. By treating and clearing the aura of energy congestion, you begin to work on the potential cause of illness before its manifestation in the body and thereby promote healing. Even after a problem has developed in the body, a client can more readily accept healing energy when the aura is treated first. Therefore, whether you are doing a partial or full energy healing treatment, scan the aura first.

There are many layers of auras surrounding our body. For our purposes we will only be dealing with the inner aura, the condition of which is indicative of a person's physical health. Be patient . . . it takes time and practice to be able to scan well. Do not judge or analyze, just try to accept exactly what comes and what impressions you receive. If you cannot feel the other person's energy or aura right away, just relax and trust that you are still able to help that individual.

The Scanning Procedure

I should mention that when doing any type of energy healing work, whether Reiki, Gentle Energy Touch, or prana work, it is important to put your tongue on the roof of your mouth just behind the hard palate (the hard ridge behind your top row of teeth). Keep it there throughout your self-healing session. This serves to connect the two major energy channels that run down the front and back of your body where your major chakras are located. Keeping your tongue on the roof of your mouth increases your sensitivity to the energy.

VERY IMPORTANT: Always scan in a downward motion, never upward, because you can cause energy blockage/congestion and/or contamination of another area in an aura that has not been cleared yet.

The first step in scanning (or any energy work) should always be to surround yourself with God's white and golden light for protection. Then call in the healing energy and say a prayer of thanks for this opportunity to help yourself or another person. You may also ask spiritually to see a mental image of what and where their problem may possibly be.

It is best to stand when scanning another person. The person you are scanning can sit, stand, or lie down as long as the position is comfortable.

Scanning is done with your arms stretched out in front of you with your hands open and palms facing the individual. As the energy flows through your hands, concentrate on the centers of your palms (hand chakras). While scanning, these hand chakras will be activated, making your hands especially sensitive to subtle energy changes and allowing you to sense and feel the other person's aura.

Stand in front of and slightly to the side of them about two to three feet away and begin to slowly walk toward the front of their body. The purpose of this is to find the outside edge of their inner aura where the scanning will be done. When you feel a tingling sensation, heat, or slight pressure in your hands, you have reached the outer edge of their inner aura.

If you do not feel their aura or energy right away, please do not get discouraged. Just move back, breathe and relax, focus, and begin again until you feel it. Once you have reached the inner aura, stretch your arms up so your hands are level with the person's head. Then begin scanning in sections (either beginning with the right front or left front of their body) in a slow and even motion, moving your hands slowly downward in front of the body all the way to their feet. Once you have scanned the front and sides of the body, walk to the back and begin scanning the same way as in the front.

Feel for areas that may be "congested" or feel "different." Congestion, in this sense, can refer to a sensation of feeling thicker, larger, fuller, or warmer than another area. It may also feel like a magnet, drawing you to a certain area or pushing against your hand.

You may also perceive the site is cooler, indented, or rippled. There may be the same tingling sensation, heat, or slight pressure on your hands you sensed when finding the outside of the aura. If any of these sensations are present, it indicates there may be a problem there. Be sure to make some mental notes of what you are feeling and where.

HOW TO INTERPRET THE RESULTS OF A SCAN

When scanning, you want to try to notice any differences in the energy field, such as an uneven shape, the absence of sensation, a sense of emptiness, or a feeling of fullness or protrusion in any area. A feeling of emptiness in an area is caused by depletion of life force energy. The surrounding meridians (energy channels that nourish and energize the whole body) may be partially or severely blocked, preventing life force energy from flowing freely and vitalizing the area.

A feeling of fullness in an area may be caused by a congestion of energy or a particular chakra being open too widely. This feeling of fullness may also be an excess of prana (life force energy) that may be leaking. If the area feels indented, a leakage of life force energy may also be present or a particular chakra may be blocked. These areas can become diseased after a certain period of time if not cleansed, balanced, and sealed.

Pay attention to what you are seeing, feeling, or hearing. Trust your awareness and your intuition. The sensations you feel in your palms—tingling, pressure, pulsation, heat, or cold—can be a clue to a problem your partner may be experiencing. You may see a certain color or feel other sensations in your hands such as denseness or a thin or thick texture.

As you interact with the energy field, you may become aware of possible personal problems or the cause of the congestion. Listening is as important as feeling because you may also be given insight intuitively on how the problems were created and what your partner can do to facilitate the healing. If you are guided to do so, share the information with them. Come from the heart and without judgment. This is sacred work. Always respect the other person's challenges and feelings.

When you are completely finished with the scanning procedure, make a mental note of the areas you found to be either depleted or congested and then proceed with the next healing technique: sweeping/clearing.

At the back of the book you will find a link to a video I created to explain how to scan and sweep/clear the aura. It also provides information on how to fill in voids, balance and ground the other person, and seal an aura.

"You think of us as beings of light and joy, which we are, but you seldom think of humans as beings of light, which you are."

—Dorothy Maclean

Sweep and Clear the Aura

Now that you've scanned the aura, it's time to clear it. Sweeping and clearing remove congested and diseased energy and cleanse, strengthen, and greatly facilitate the healing process. Many simple illnesses can be healed just by sweeping and clearing the aura. I recommend sweeping/clearing a person's energy field at the beginning of every Gentle Energy Touch session.

Our auras and chakras are like magnets, picking up vibration energy from the environment (including the energies of other people, whether positive or negative). These energies are then distributed throughout the physical body, which in turn, sends energies outward via the chakras to the aura. This is an ongoing process of receiving energies and emitting energies.

When sweeping your own or someone else's energy field, your concentration and intention should be to cleanse the aura of any diseased/negative energy that may have gotten attached. This technique will make a Gentle Energy Touch session more effective. Even though you are not actually touching the physical body while sweeping the aura fields, sweeping heals and balances those fields that directly affect physical health.

Once again, begin by surrounding yourself and the person you are doing a session on with white light for protection before calling for healing energy. Say a prayer giving thanks for this opportunity to help another person and for that person's return to good health. If you have called for energy prior to scanning, then it is not necessary to call it in again. (See page pp. 89-91, "Ask for Divine Healing Energy.")

The person you are working on can choose to sit in a chair, stand, or lie down while you sweep the aura. Any position is appropriate as long as your partner is comfortable. Healing is a lot easier if a person is relaxed and receptive. It is important not to have any expectations about the outcome of the treatment. Remember it is your partner's healing, and it is that person's choice to accept it or not.

PROCEDURE FOR SWEEPING

Your hands and fingers are used in sweeping and clearing the aura. Basically there are two hand positions: one is a cupped-hand position facing upward to receive the energy, and the other is a spread-finger position that is the same as putting your hand into a baseball glove. The spread-finger position is effective in the removal of diseased energy, and is also utilized in combing and straightening/smoothing out the area after you have removed the diseased energy with the same hand. It doesn't matter which hand you use. The spread-finger hand will sweep/clear down, while the cupped hand is turned upward. If the healer does not concentrate on one receiving hand (one turned upward), the healer may become easily exhausted since they tend to use their own energy instead of Divine energy.

Begin by sweeping/combing through the aura surrounding the body from head to toe. Place your hand a few inches above the physical body and slowly sweep through the aura with fingers spread. Do this for the front as well as the back of the body. If you feel dense or heavy areas, then sweep the area for a few moments until you feel the area is beginning to clear. Keep in mind that when you scanned the aura before you made mental notes of where there might be congestion. Just a note here: while I sweep and clear the aura with my spread-fingered hand, I visualize that hand is like a spiderweb, catching all the congested energy into it.

As you clear the diseased/congested energy from the aura or chakras, visualize a fire or a bucket filled with green or orange flames on the ground beside you and constantly throw all the congested energies into the fire/bucket. This will prevent any accumulation of unwanted energy next to you. Be very careful not to step on this area of discarded energy since you might pick it up into your own aura. When your sweeping is complete, make sure you put out the fire. Simply visualize the fire or bucket of energy being extinguished with healing water and send those energies seeping into Mother Earth with love, light, and healing.

Then scan the aura again to be sure that the unwanted energies have been removed. Learn to use and trust your intuition.

It is important to fill the areas that you have cleared of unwanted energies with God's healing white light. Use a clockwise motion with the palm of your right or left hand as you visualize this white healing light pouring into the areas where you removed energies. The white healing light will heal, protect, and energize the area. This should be done after you have completed your scanning, sweeping, and healing session. If you are doing only scanning and sweeping, then make sure you fill in the areas with God's light when that is done.

THINGS TO AVOID WHEN SCANNING AND SWEEPING

Do not apply too much sweeping energy on infants, very young children, the very weak, or the elderly. The chakras of infants and very young children are not as strong as those of adults and can easily be overenergized and become congested. The chakras of very weak and/or elderly patients are similarly fragile. Sweeping a weak aura can result in a choking effect on the chakras. This is similar to the choking reaction of a very thirsty person who drinks too much water in too short a time. Weakened and older people are slow to assimilate prana. They should be scanned, swept, and cleared gently, gradually, and over a period of time. They should also be allowed to rest and assimilate prana for about fifteen to twenty minutes before being swept again, or stop the sweeping and begin healing with Gentle Energy Touch (see pp. 118-172 for positions).

Important Notes

- Never sweep the heart from the front. The heart is quite sensitive and delicate and must be swept from the back and not for a long period of time. Too much sweeping may cause the heart to beat faster than it normally does.

- Do not sweep/clear the eyes directly. The eyes are very delicate like the heart, and you can easily cause congestion in that area. The eyes should be swept/cleared from the back of the head and not for a long period of time.

- Always sweep in a downward motion; never sweep in an upward motion. Sweeping upward will cause the body to become contaminated with congested energy.

Please know that prana scanning/sweeping/clearing is quite safe as long as you properly follow the given guidelines and instructions.

"Today a new sun rises for me; everything lives, everything is animated, everything seems to speak to me of my passion, everything invites me to cherish it."

—ANNE LENCLOS

CHAPTER 7

Gentle Energy Touch Self-Healing Positions

Now that you've swept the aura, you are ready to move on to the healing positions. This first set is composed of positions to use in your own self-healing treatments. Refer to the description for information on what each can be used for. In chapter 10, I'll tell you how to balance the chakras, fill in voids with God's healing light, ground yourself to Mother Earth, close your aura to keep healing energies in your body, and disconnect from the healing energy to end a session. Reading through all these sections prior to doing a self-healing will let you know what to expect and makes for a smoother treatment flow.

Each position should be held for approximately two to three minutes, but if you feel the need to stay at a position longer, do so. Do not rush your session. You should truly do all of the positions daily for at least for twenty-one days, and then trust in your inner knowing of what feels comfortable for you thereafter. Remember, it takes approximately twenty-one days to balance all of the chakras. But after that, please do not stop doing your healing; continuing this gift on approximately a weekly basis will bring continued benefits.

POSITION 1 *(Seventh Chakra—Crown)*

Gently place both hands on the top of the head with finger-tips slightly touching.

This position may be helpful for spiritual awakening, "seeing" the whole picture, inspiration, devotion, purposefulness, and being ethical.

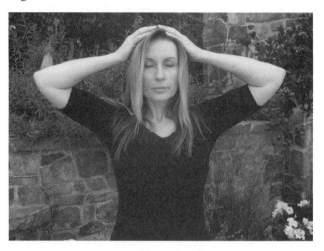

POSITION 2 *(Sixth Chakra—Third Eye)*

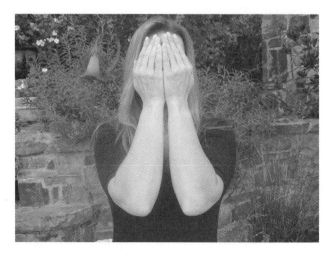

Gently place your hands side by side, palms facing you, in front of your face, covering the forehead, eyes, nose, and cheekbones.

This position may be associated with wisdom, "seeing" a clearer picture, dealing with reality, improving psychic abilities, resolution of anger, or mental acuity.

POSITION 3

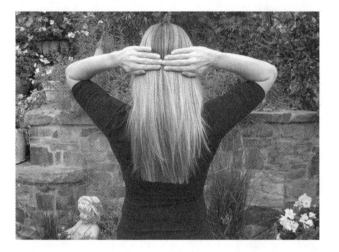

Place both of your hands at the back of your head with fingertips slightly touching.

This position may promote peacefulness, balance, confidence in being yourself, and self-appreciation.

POSITION 4

Place your **right** hand over your right ear and your **left** hand over your left ear.

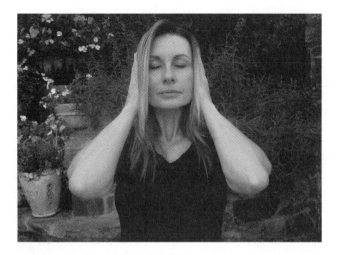

This position may be helpful for hearing your inner voice, being amenable to listening to others, or open-mindedness.

POSITION 5 *(Fifth Chakra—Throat)*

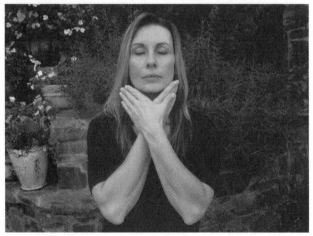

Spread your right thumb and index finger and cup your throat with your **right** hand. Take your **left** hand, spreading your thumb and index finger, and place it along your lower jawline, resting it just above your right hand.

This position promotes ability to speak your mind, release anger, the flow of your creativity, and accepting change.

POSITION 6 *(Fourth Chakra—Heart)*

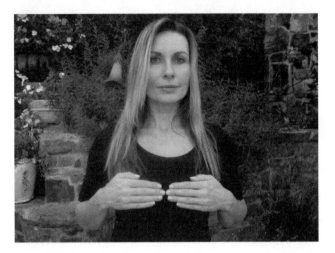

Place both of your hands horizontally on the chest area with your fingertips slightly touching.

This position promotes self-love, love of others, and a passion for life, loyalty, tranquility, optimism, and peacefulness.

POSITION 7 *(Third Chakra—Solar Plexus)*

Place both of your hands horizontally at the base (bottom) of the rib cage with your fingertips touching.

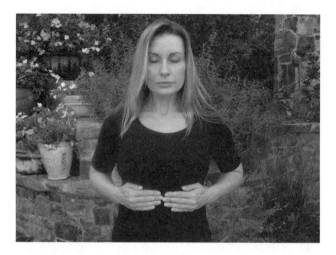

This position is helpful for peace of mind, inner calmness, strength of character, or love of self and others. It promotes self-confidence, self-respect, your ability to handle a crisis, and flexibility.

POSITION 8 *(Second Chakra—Sacral)*

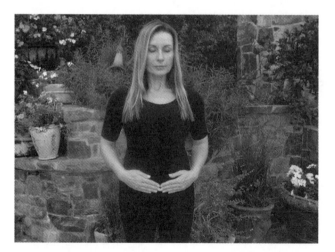

Place both of your hands on the lower abdomen area below your navel.

This position is associated with letting go of past issues and controlling others, decisiveness, acceptance of love, or confidence in money and sexual matters.

POSITION 9 *(First Chakra—Root)*

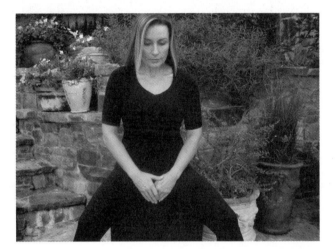

Cup both of your hands, place the **right** hand over the **left** hand and place both over your pubic area.

The position is helpful for resolving family issues, letting go of past belief systems, feeling free, loyalty, and acceptance.

All of the following leg positions are useful in promoting standing your ground in life, being flexible, moving forward with decisions, and standing up for yourself and others. They are also helpful for arthritic pain, leg injuries, and circulation.

POSITION 10

Place both of your hands side by side, palms down, on the upper outer right thigh area. Place your **right** hand first, with your **left** hand next to your right hand.

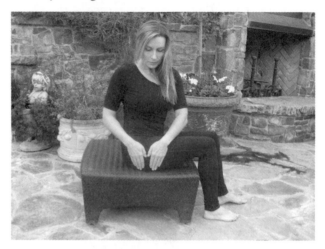

POSITION 11

Cup both of your hands and place them on top of your right knee.

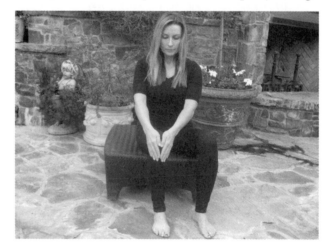

POSITION 12

Place both of your hands around the middle of the right lower leg, cupping your **right** hand in the back at the base of the calf and your **left** hand parallel to the right in the front.

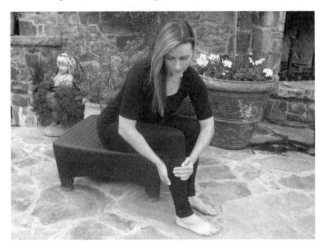

POSITION 13

Continue down to your right ankle area, cupping the **right** hand in back of the ankle and the **left** hand in the front of the ankle.

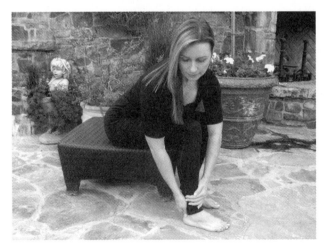

POSITION 14

"Run the energy" from the sole of your right foot to the right hip by placing your **right** hand on your right hip and your **left** hand on the bottom of your right foot.

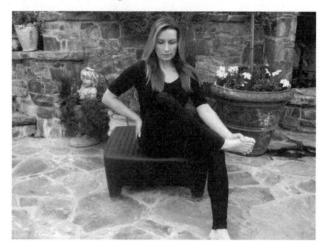

VERY IMPORTANT: You have now completed your right side. Follow **POSITIONS 10 through 14** by running through the same positions for the left side, reversing the hands, placing your left first and then your right, then proceed to **POSITION 15**.

POSITION 15

Place your **right** hand over your **right** foot and your **left** hand over your **left** foot.

Visualize or ask God to fill all the areas where energy was released with white healing light. We do not want to leave any voids.

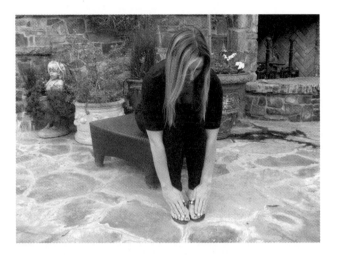

BALANCING THE CHAKRAS, GROUNDING, CLOSING THE AURA, AND DISCONNECTING THE ENERGY

End every Gentle Energy Healing touch session with the steps of balancing the chakras, grounding, closing the aura, giving thanks, and disconnecting from the healing energy. All of these processes are described in chapter 10.

This will complete your treatment.

Optional Self-Healing Positions

The Universal and individual leg positions are optional. I use the Universal Position many times if I begin to feel stress and need to balance myself quickly no matter where I may be. It is quick and takes just a few seconds to do. I set my intention to connect myself back to my heart with love and compassion and to my solar plexus for getting back into my personal power. It provides me with a feeling of happiness and gratefulness. I become more thankful for what life provides and remember never to take things for granted.

POSITION 16

One more position you'll want to learn is the Universal Position. It is a quick fix for balancing, centering, and loving. Place your **left** hand on your heart and your **right** hand on your solar plexus. This position can be used after you have completed your self-healing session and anytime you feel the need to become balanced and centered.

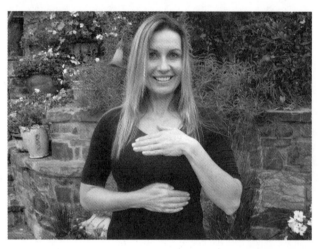

It's a great "I love and I am happy with myself" position.

The leg positions beginning on the following page show a different way of healing your legs. When I had arthritis, I did healing on one leg at a time, and I felt this was very beneficial because the pain varied in each leg. If your legs have no physical challenges, then doing both at the same time is shorter, or you may find it okay to skip your legs completely. However, you still must ground and balance yourself. Do what feels right for you.

LEG POSITIONS

You can do both legs at the same time or individually—whichever you find easier for you. If you are experiencing joint or leg pain, I suggest doing your legs individually.

Treatment in these areas promotes confidence in moving forward, flexibility with life's situations, a proper pace with activity, the ability to change direction, feeling grounded, and sure-footedness. It may help with leg and arthritis pain.

POSITION 17

Place your **right** hand on your right thigh and your **left** hand on your left thigh.

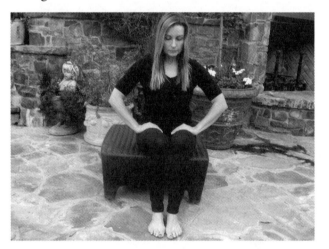

POSITION 18

Place your **right** hand on your right knee and your **left** hand on
your left knee.

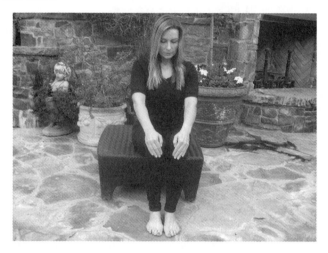

POSITION 19

Place your **right** hand on your right shin and your **left** hand on
your left shin.

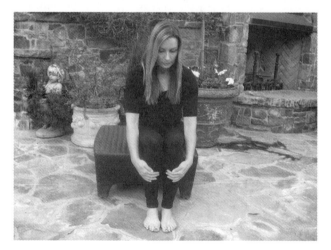

POSITION 20

Place your **right** hand on your right ankle and your **left** hand on your left ankle.

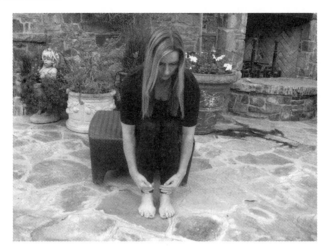

POSITION 21

This is for balancing the chakras, grounding, closing the aura, and disconnecting the energy.

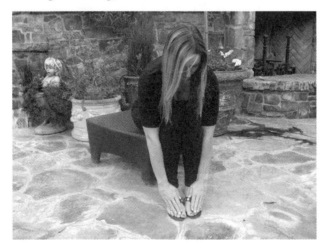

Place your **right** hand on your right foot and your **left** hand on your left foot and proceed to balance the chakras as described in chapter 10, followed by grounding, closing the aura, giving thanks, and disconnecting.

This will complete your treatment.

CHAPTER 8

Gentle Energy Touch
Table Positions

*"The Self is not something ready-made, but something in
continuous formation through choice of action."*
—JOHN DEWEY

You do not necessarily need to do all the table positions noted
here, but it is important to make sure you do a healing on all of
the seven chakras. When you have completed the seven chakras,
then go back to where you intuitively feel the other person needs
healing. The receiver may also have expressed where they are hurt-
ing prior to the session. So go back and apply more energy healing and/or clearing to the areas where there are challenges. Many
of the positions help the receiver to release stress, relax, and feel
peaceful. The shoulder and hand positions help them to feel loved.
Each position should be held for approximately two to three minutes. If you feel the need to stay longer on an area, do so. Do not
rush a session!

Important: When doing healing positions, do not slide your
hands. Lift your hands to the next position.

POSITION 1 *(Seventh Chakra—Crown)*

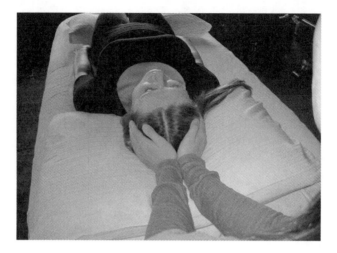

Gently place the palms of your hands on the crown of the head with your hands resting gently on the sides of the skull and the fingers pointing toward the ears. This area is associated with the skull; the brain, including part of the frontal lobe, the parietal and temporal lobes, the cerebrum, the hypothalamus, pituitary, and pineal glands and the bodily functions they control; and the ears. Problems in this area may be associated with brain tumors, headaches, strokes, head injuries, seizures, muscular and skeletal difficulties, stress/chronic exhaustion not linked to physical disorders, hearing difficulties, and sensitivity to sound, light, and the environment.

POSITION 2 *(Sixth Chakra—Crown)*

Cup both hands over the forehead, eyes, and nose with your fingertips at the region of the upper teeth. This area is associated with the brain, including the frontal lobe, the pituitary and hypothalamus glands and the bodily functions they control. This area is also associated with the sinuses, eyes, nose, and upper jaw and teeth. Blockage here may be the source of such difficulties as nervous system disorders, brain tumors, seizures, headaches, sinusitis, eye disorders, jaw and upper teeth complaints, fatigue, stress, and colds. Relaxing the eyes helps to relax the entire body.

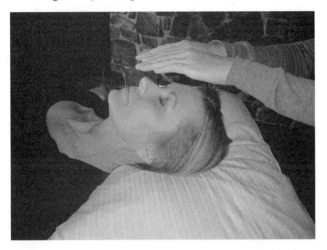

POSITION 3

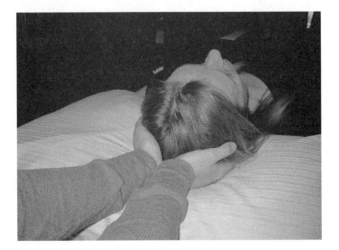

Gently place your hands at the back of the head, cradling the skull in the palms of your hands. The outside edges of your hands are touching and the fingertips are at the base of the skull. This area is associated with the occipital lobe of the brain, the cerebellum and the brain stem and the bodily functions they control, the skull, upper cervical vertebrae, and the ears. Blockage here may be the source of such difficulties as seizures or strokes; problems with balance, vision, hearing, sleep and waking states; tension; and headaches.

POSITION 4 *(Fifth Chakra—Throat)*

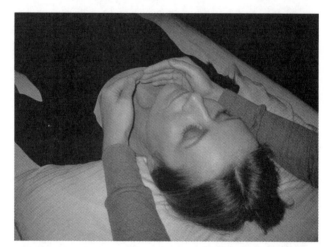

Cup both of your hands with fingertips touching around the throat area (but not on the actual throat), staying near the chin line. This area is associated with the neck, including the cervical vertebrae, spinal cord, larynx, thyroid and parathyroid glands and the bodily functions they control, carotid arteries, tonsils, lower jaw, and teeth. Blockage here may be the source of such difficulties as nerve impingement affecting the arms and hands and/or other parts of the body, laryngitis, vocal cord problems, sore throat, swollen glands, tonsillitis, gum or tooth problems, swallowing difficulty, metabolic problems, or difficulty with communication.

POSITION 5

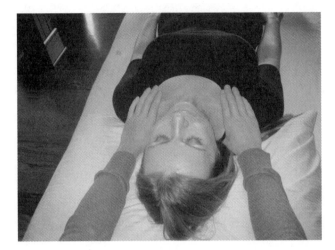

Gently lay your hands on top of the shoulders, thumbs down toward the receiver's back. This area is associated with the upper ribs, collarbone, upper shoulder blades, upper cervical nerves, and muscles that may affect the arms and hands. Problems in this area may be associated with a pinched cervical nerve or tightness of the muscles from stress or injury. This position is very soothing and helps to calm the receiver, relieving stress and/or anxieties. In this position, notice when the receiver lets go of any shoulder tension.

POSITION 6

Gently place your hands under the shoulder blades with fingers pointing toward the mid-back. This area is associated with the shoulders, shoulder blades and muscles, cervical and thoracic nerves innervating the shoulders, arms, and upper ribs. Difficulties in this area may be associated with shoulder and arm pain, stiffness, and numbness or tingling of the arms/hands. I have found this position most helpful for upper back and shoulder pain and for relaxing and calming the receiver.

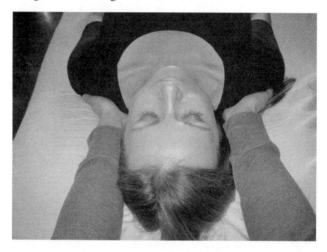

POSITION 7

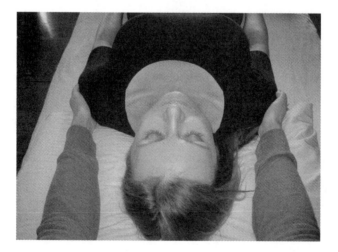

Gently place your hands under the upper arms, fingers pointing toward the elbows. This area is associated with the muscles, nerves, and bones in the shoulders, arms, and hands. Problems in this area may be associated with arthritis and shoulder, arm, or hand pain or numbness. I have found this position most useful for relaxing and calming the receiver. People often express a feeling of security when I do this position.

POSITION 8 *(Fourth Chakra—Heart)*

Stand at the receiver's right side and place your hands gently on the upper chest. Place your **left** hand on their right side and your **right** hand on their left side. Or you can position both hands hovering one to two inches above instead of touching these areas. This position is associated with the ribs, upper thoracic vertebrae and nerves, esophagus, thymus gland, lymph system, lungs, trachea, heart, spinal cord, and muscles. Problems in this area may be associated with rib or vertebrae fractures, back pain, difficulty swallowing, immune system deficiencies, lung conditions, difficulty breathing, pneumonia, bronchitis, heart conditions, and nerve disorders.

POSITION 9A *(Fourth Chakra—Heart)*

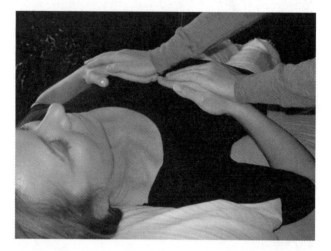

This position should be discussed with women prior to treatment. In most cases, I gently place their hands over the breast area and then place my hands over their hands. This area is associated with the breasts, lungs, heart, ribs and mid-thoracic vertebrae, and spinal cord. Difficulties in this area may be associated with breast disorders/cancer, lung disease, heart conditions, rib and/or vertebrae fracture or deterioration, and nerve disorders.

POSITION 9B *(Fourth Chakra—Heart)*

If position 9A was not discussed with the woman prior to treatment, you can use this alternative hand position. Position both hands hovering one to two inches above the breast area. This allows for effective treatment without touching the receiver inappropriately.

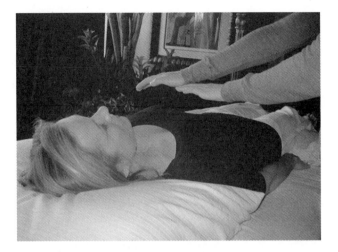

POSITION 10 *(Third Chakra—Solar Plexus)*

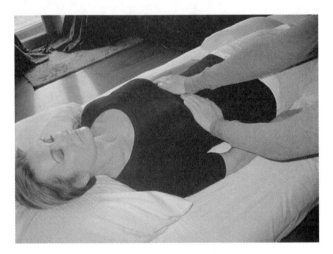

Gently place both hands below the breast area over the rib cage. This area is associated with the ribs, lower thoracic vertebrae and nerves, spinal cord, diaphragm, lower lungs, esophagus, stomach, spleen, pancreas, liver, gallbladder, abdominal aorta, and part of the small and large intestines. This may be the locale of such difficulties as rib or vertebrae fractures, nerve disorders, hiccups, asthma, pneumonia, digestion problems, ulcers, diabetes/blood sugar irregularities, pancreatitis, hepatitis, gallbladder disease, intestinal difficulties, and circulatory problems in the abdomen and/or legs.

POSITION 11 *(Third Chakra—Solar Plexus)*

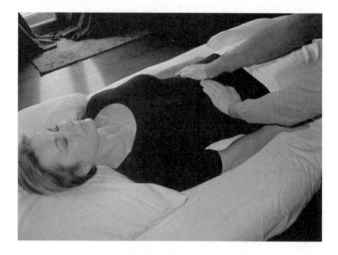

Do not slide your hands to any of the positions. Lift your hands from Position 10 and gently place them on the middle abdomen toward the end of the rib cage. This area is associated with the small and large intestines; lower thoracic/lumbar vertebrae, nerves, and muscles; lower portion of the spinal cord; ribs; liver; pancreas; stomach; gallbladder; kidneys; adrenal glands; and abdominal aorta. Problems in this area may be associated with digestive disorders, elimination difficulties, mid and lower back pain, kidney disease, adrenal imbalance, and circulation difficulties in the abdomen/legs.

POSITION 12 *(Second Chakra—Sacral)*

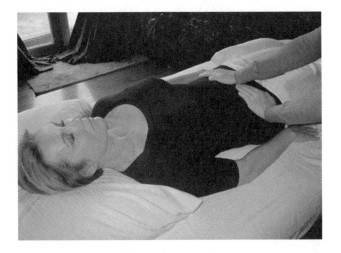

Gently continue down the front of the body. Do not slide your hands to this next position. Lift your hands and place them on the lower abdomen between the hip bones and below the waist. This area is associated with the small and large intestines, the bladder, reproductive organs, and lower lumbar and sacral vertebrae, nerves, and muscles. Difficulties in this area may be associated with elimination disorders (intestinal or urinary), pregnancy/menstruation difficulties, lower back pain, and poor circulation/pain in the legs.

POSITION 13 *(First Chakra—Root)*

Position your hands hovering approximately two inches above the pubic bone and genitalia. This area is associated with the lower sacral/coccyx vertebrae, nerves, and muscles, as well as the pelvis, reproductive organs, bladder, prostate, and rectum. Blockages here may be the source of such difficulties as pain in the lower back and legs, problems with the reproductive organs/prostate, and elimination problems with the intestines or bladder.

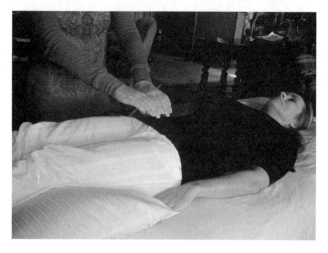

POSITION 14

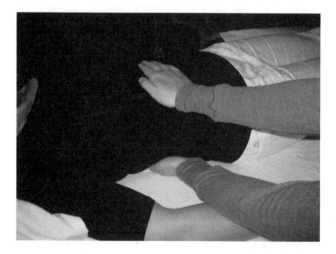

When treating the right side, place your **right** hand on the belly, just above the waist, and your **left** hand on their back, just below the rib cage (on top of the kidneys). This area is associated with the kidneys, adrenal glands, lower thoracic/lumbar vertebrae, liver, and small and large intestines. Difficulties in this area may present with urinary difficulties/infection, allergies, back pain, or digestion/elimination difficulties. This position may be helpful for adrenal gland problems, kidney disorders, lower back pain, abdominal pain, diabetes, allergies, and stress. Those having a healing session find this very soothing.

POSITION 15

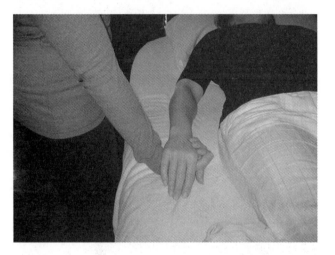

Gently take the receiver's hand into yours, palm to palm, thumbs interlocking. This area is associated with the hand, arm, elbow, shoulder, neck, muscles, and cervical and thoracic nerves and vertebrae. Problems in this area may be associated with pain/difficulties in the neck, shoulder, arm, and/or hand.

POSITION 16

While maintaining your **right** hand position, palm to palm, gently place your **left** hand on top of the receiver's hand. For areas associated with this position, see Position 15.

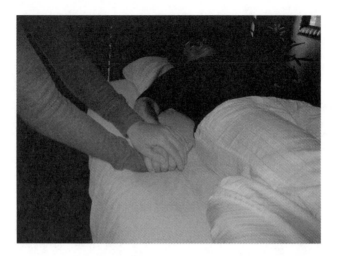

People have told me that this position felt very comforting and nurturing to them.

POSITION 17

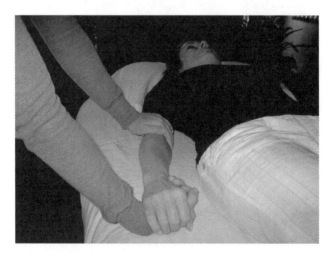

This position is called **"running the energy"** from the **HAND** to the **ELBOW**. Maintain Position 16 with your **right** hand and the receiver's palm to palm and place your **left** hand on top of the elbow area. This position may help to remove any blocked energy in the arm and is useful for the areas of association discussed in Position 15.

POSITION 18

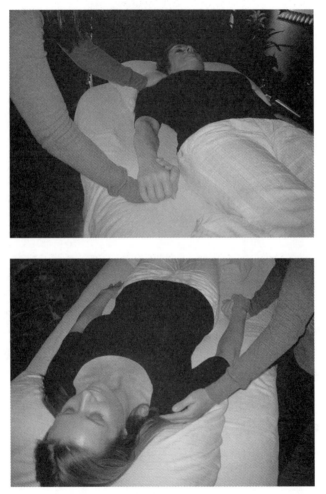

This position is called **"running the energy"** from the **HAND** to the **SHOULDER**. Maintain Position 16 with your **right** hand and the receiver's palm to palm and place your **left** hand on the shoulder. This may be useful for releasing blocked energy and stress as well as for conditions associated with this area as noted in Position 15.

POSITION 19

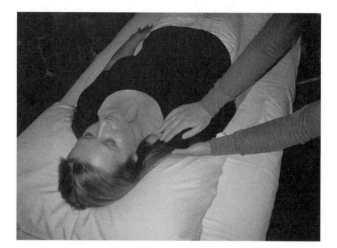

After running the energy from the hand to the shoulder in Position 18, cup the shoulder front and back with both hands. This area is associated with the shoulder, neck, muscles, cervical/thoracic nerves, arm, and hand. Difficulties in this area may be associated with neck, shoulder, arm, or hand pain/numbness. This position can be a very soothing and relaxing one.

POSITION 20 through POSITION 28 are useful for problems associated with the legs, knees, and feet.

POSITION 20

Gently place the right hand of the receiver on their abdomen. Place both of your hands side by side with your fingers together on the side of the right hip and upper thigh area. This area is associated with the bones in the hip, thigh, knee, and foot; lumbar/sacral nerves and muscles; and blood flow through the leg. Blockages here may be associated with such difficulties as pain in the hip, lower back, leg, knee, or foot and circulatory problems from the thigh to the foot.

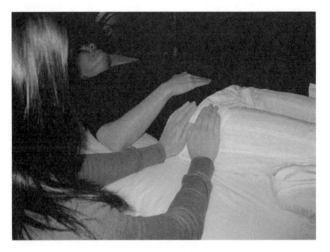

POSITION 21

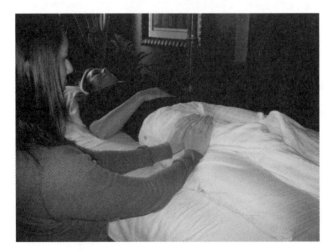

Gently continue down the thigh by moving to the next lower position adjacent to the previous area, keeping both hands together and lifting the hands for each new position.

POSITION 22

Gently continue down the thigh area, keeping both hands together and lifting the hands for placement in this new position. Put your hands on the top of the thigh above the right knee.

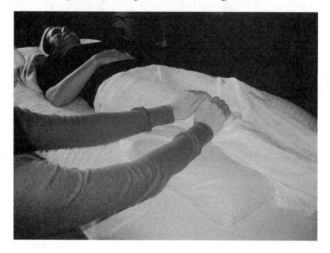

POSITION 23

Cup the knee with both hands, placing your **right** hand on top of your partner's right knee and your **left** hand under the knee. Hold firmly but gently.

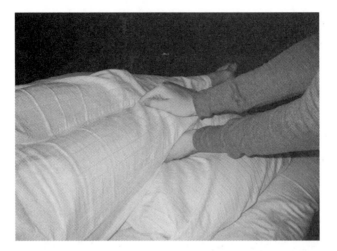

POSITION 24

Gently continue down to the lower leg area, placing your hands on the right shin midway between the knee and the ankle, keeping both hands together, and lifting the hands for this new position.

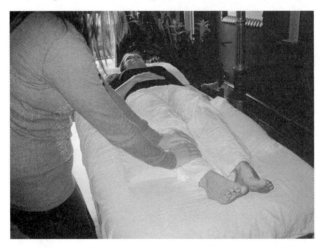

POSITION 25

Cup the ankle with your hands, placing your **left** hand under and your **right** hand over the ankle or along each side of the ankle. Hold firmly but gently.

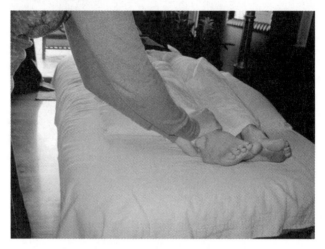

POSITION 26

Run the energy up the leg from the **ANKLE** to the **KNEE**. Keep your **right** hand on top of the ankle and place your **left** hand on the knee.

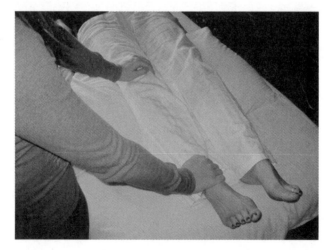

POSITION 27

Now run the energy up the leg from the **ANKLE** to the **HIP**. Keep your **right** hand on the ankle and place your **left** hand on the hip.

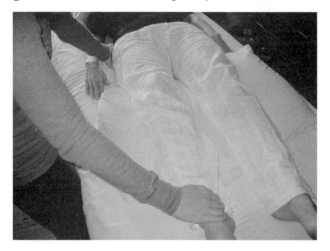

POSITION 28

Now run the energy up the leg from the **SOLE OF THE FOOT** to the **HIP.** Place your **right** hand on the bottom of the receiver's right foot and your **left** hand on the side of the hip.

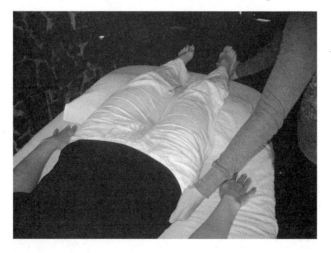

All of the "run the energy" positions (**POSITIONS 17, 18, 26, 27, and 28**) will work to boost the immune system of the person being healed. Running the energy through the bones of the arms and legs sends positive and strengthening energy flowing throughout the entire body. This helps the body feel whole and energized.

You are now finished on the right side of the person. Do not cross over to their other side by way of the feet. Walk back up to the head before moving over to the left side. At this point, the treatment may have already released blocked energy that will now be flowing outward by way of the feet and hands, and this outpouring should not be impeded. Set your intention to send any energies that are at the feet down to Mother Earth with love and light and healing. If you should step below the feet by accident, the unwanted energies will have been sent away by your intention so you will not get contaminated. Now proceed to the left side.

START the left side treatment with POSITION 14 reversing your hand positions. NOW REPEAT POSITIONS 15 THROUGH 28. When you are finished, proceed to POSITION 29.

POSITION 29

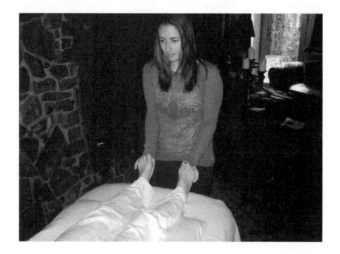

After you have completed working on the left side, you are ready to begin "closing down" or finishing the treatment. Stand at the feet of the person being healed and gently lay your hands on the soles of the feet. **See the complete instructions for balancing, grounding, closing the aura, and disconnecting energy in chapter 10.**

POSITIONS 29A and 29B

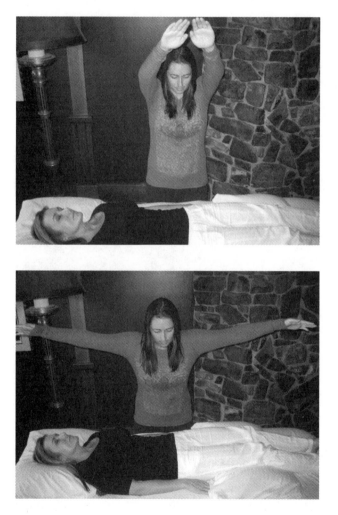

Positions 29A and 29B illustrate the hand positions for closing the aura.

Back Positions

After you have balanced, grounded, and closed the aura, gently rouse the receiver from the restful, relaxed state of the healing—or from sleep if necessary—and let them know it is time to sit up. Then proceed with the following positions if this person has been experiencing back or neck pain.

POSITION 30

Gently lay both of your hands on the receiver's shoulders. This position releases tension in the shoulders and relieves headaches from tense neck and shoulder muscles. This shoulder position can be very comforting.

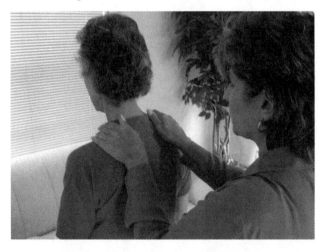

POSITION 31

Gently place both of your hands on the shoulder blades. This position is useful for treating the shoulder muscles, stress, and anxiety and can be very relaxing.

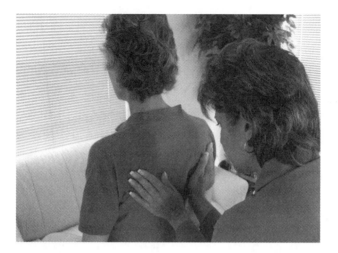

POSITION 32

Gently place both of your hands with palms facing out on the lower back just above the waist and over the adrenal area. This position is associated with the adrenal glands that are very often weakened by our stressful lifestyles. This position can be very relaxing and comforting.

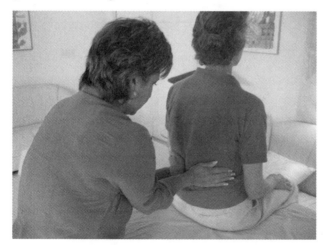

POSITION 33

Place your **right** hand at the base of the neck and your **left** hand at the end of the spine area on the lower back. This position runs the energy **UP THE SPINE** to the **BASE OF THE NECK**, which sends positive and strengthening energy flowing throughout the entire body. The body will now feel connected and energized.

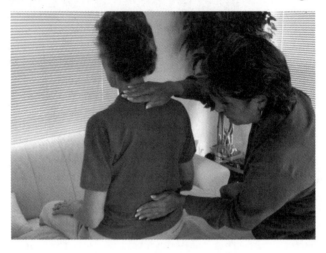

Optional Table Positions

Since people may fall asleep during the treatment and do not like lying on their stomach, I do not wake someone I am working on and have them turn over to complete the twelve back positions. As I do the treatment at the front, by setting my intention, I also address the energy of the back positions as I work my way down the body. If, however, you wish to have the receiver turn over onto their stomach, and that is okay for your partner, follow the **Optional Table Positions 34 thru 44.**

POSITION 34 *(Seventh Chakra—Crown)*

Gently place both hands side by side at the top of the head. Fingers should be together with the thumbs touching. The heels of both hands should be toward the front of the receiver's skull and the fingers should be facing the back of the skull.

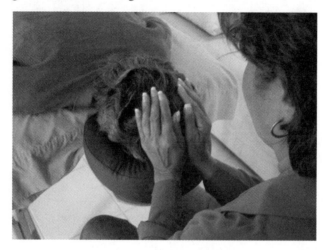

This area is associated with the skull; the brain, including part of the frontal lobe, the parietal and temporal lobes, the cerebrum, the hypothalamus, pituitary, and pineal glands and the bodily functions they control; and the ears. Problems in this area may be associated with brain tumors, headaches, strokes, head injuries, seizures, muscular and skeletal difficulties, and stress, chronic exhaustion not linked to physical disorders, hearing difficulties, and sensitivity to sound, light, and the environment. This position can be helpful for tension, headaches, anxiety, and calming emotions such as fear.

POSITION 35

Gently place both hands on the back of the head with the fingers together pointing down toward the base of the skull and thumbs touching.

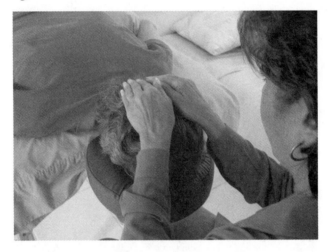

This area is associated with the occipital lobe of the brain, the cerebellum and the brain stem and the bodily functions they control, the skull, the upper cervical vertebrae, and the ears. This area may be the locale of such difficulties as seizures, strokes, and problems with balance, vision, hearing, sleep and arousal state, tension, headaches, and anxiety. Applying this hand position calms the mind and the emotions.

POSITION 36

Gently place both hands on top of the shoulder area at the base of the neck with fingers pointing together toward the spine.

This area is associated with the shoulders, shoulder blades and muscles, cervical and thoracic nerves innervating the shoulders and arms, and upper ribs. Difficulties in this area may be associated with shoulder and arm pain, stiffness, or numbness and/or tingling of the arms/hands.

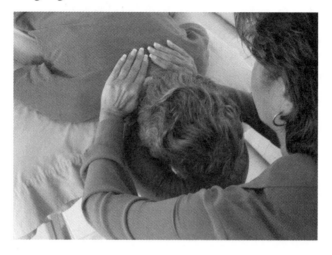

I have found this position most helpful for upper back and shoulder pain and for relaxing and calming the receiver. This releases tension in the shoulders and relieves headaches caused by tension in the neck and shoulder muscles.

POSITION 37

Moving to your **RIGHT** around the table (to the left side of the person on the table), gently place both your hands on the shoulder blades. Place your **left** hand on their left side and your **right** hand on their right side.

This area is associated with the shoulders, ribs, upper thoracic vertebrae and nerves, lungs, and spinal cord and muscles. Problems in this area may be associated with rib or vertebrae fractures, back pain, lung conditions, difficulty breathing, and nerve disorders.

This position is useful for treating shoulder muscles and aches, stress, and anxiety and can be very relaxing.

POSITION 38

Gently place both of your hands end to end across the middle of the back area with the heels of your hands nearest you and the fingers pointing away.

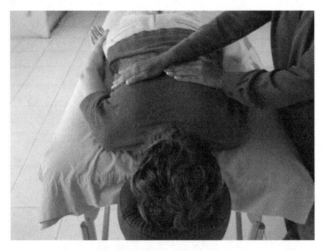

This area is associated with the ribs, lower thoracic vertebrae and nerves, spinal cord, diaphragm, lower lungs, and abdominal aorta. It may be the locale of such difficulties as rib or vertebrae fractures, back and shoulder complaints, nerve disorders, lung disorders such as asthma and pneumonia, hiccups, and circulatory problems in the abdomen. This position can also be very relaxing and soothing.

POSITION 39

Gently place both your hands on the back just above the waist and over the adrenal area using the same hand alignment as in Position 38 above.

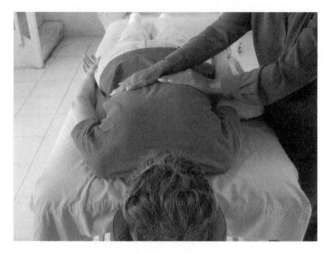

This area is associated with the lower thoracic/lumbar vertebrae, nerves, and muscles; the lower portion of the spinal cord; ribs; kidneys; adrenal glands; and abdominal aorta. Problems in this area may be associated with mid and lower back pain, kidney disease, adrenal imbalance, and circulatory difficulties in the abdomen/legs. This position is useful due to our stressful lives, which cause the adrenals to almost always be in a weakened state. This position can be rejuvenating and balancing.

POSITION 40

Place your **left** hand at the base of the neck and your **right** hand on the lower back area, fingers parallel, facing the right side of the receiver.

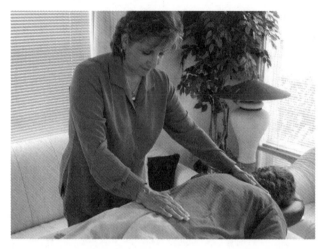

This position runs the energy from the **LOWER BACK** area to the **BASE OF THE NECK**.

Again, running the energy throughout the back area sends positive and strengthening energy flowing throughout the entire body. This treatment helps the body feel whole and energized.

POSITIONS 41 through 44 are useful for problems with the legs, knees, and feet. Use these positions for joint difficulties, sports injuries, arthritis, and any blockages affecting the flow of energy through the leg area.

POSITION 41

Gently place both of your hands on the backs of the receiver's knees: your **left** hand for the left knee and **right** hand for the right knee.

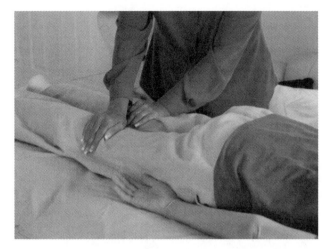

POSITION 42

Gently place your **right** hand on the left ankle of the receiver while keeping your **left** hand on the back of the left knee.

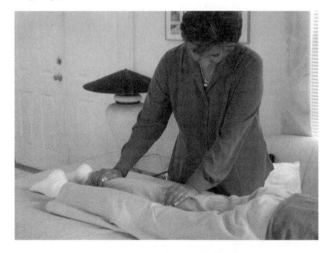

This position runs the energy up the leg from **ANKLE** to the **KNEE.**

POSITION 43

Keep your **right** hand on the left ankle and place your **left** hand on the outside of the left hip.

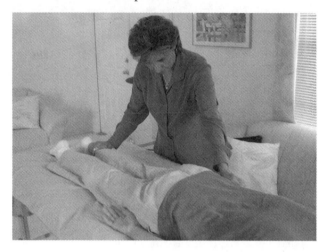

This position runs the energy up the leg from **ANKLE** to the **HIP.**

POSITION 44

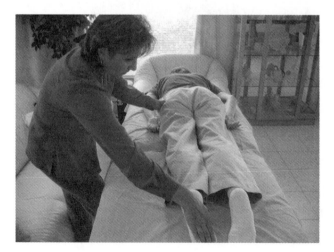

This position runs the energy up from the **SOLE OF THE FOOT (SOLE)** to the **HIP**. Keep your **left** hand on the hip area and place your **right** hand on the sole of the left foot. Remember to cross over by way of the head.

IMPORTANT NOTE: When **POSITIONS 42, 43, 44** are completed, move to the right leg and repeat them. When you switch sides, you can use whatever hand is more comfortable for you to work with.

POSITION 45

After you have completely worked on the entire body, front and back, of the receiver, begin "closing down" or finishing the treatment. Make sure you fill in all the areas where energy was released with God's healing light first. Then stand near the receiver's feet, off to the side as shown, and gently lay your hands on the soles of the feet. Proceed to balance the chakras, ground, close the aura, and disconnect the energy as detailed in chapter 10.

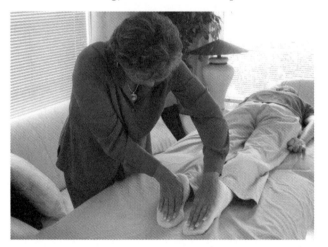

CHAPTER 9

Gentle Energy Touch
Chair Positions

If a massage table is not available, then a chair can be used for a session instead. Please note that you may begin at the left or right side using either your left or right hand. The pictures specify a hand and side, but please use the hand or side most comfortable for you.

POSITION 1 *(Seventh Chakra—Crown)*

Have the receiver sit comfortably on a chair with arms and legs uncrossed and hands resting on the thighs. Suggest for the receiver to close their eyes. Then begin your treatment.

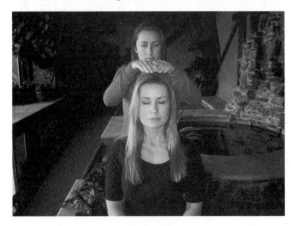

Place both hands with fingers together and thumbs touching about an inch over the crown of the head.

Difficulties in this area may be associated with feelings of inadequacy, fear of being judged, lack of purpose, loss of identity, lack of trust, selfishness, narrow-mindedness, difficulties with spirituality, depression, apathy, and confusion.

POSITION 2

Stand to the **right or left** of the receiver and place your **right** or left hand near the forehead and your **left** or right hand at the back of the neck.

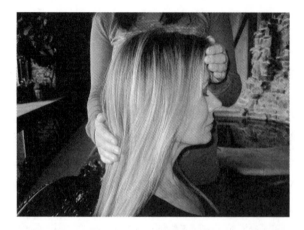

Problems may manifest in this area due to the suppression of our true dreams or desires, loss of control, stubbornness in thinking, fear of decision-making, perpetual worrying, and conflict between our intellect and our natural urges. This position is helpful in relieving worry and also tension in the neck.

POSITION 3A *(Sixth Chakra—Third Eye)*

Stand behind the receiver and position your hands, side by side with thumbs touching and fingers together pointing down, hovering in front of the receiver's face (without touching the face), covering the forehead, eyes, and nose.

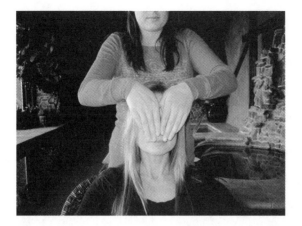

A healing touch here may be helpful for difficulties with fear or phobias concerning the future, reality problems, psychic difficulties, repressed anger, and resistance to dealing with some situation or person.

POSITION 3B *(Alternate to 3A)*

Place both hands horizontally with fingertips touching in front of the receiver's face (without touching the face), covering the eyes, nose, upper cheeks, and temple areas.

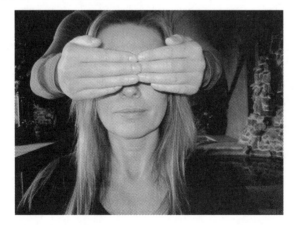

Difficulties in this area may be associated with repressed self-expression, fear of making the wrong decisions, inability to act on achieving your desires, or a blockage between the material and the spiritual world.

POSITION 4

Stand behind the receiver and lightly place both hands on the tops of the shoulders.

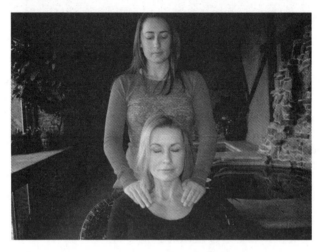

Problems in this area may manifest due to feeling emotionally burdened, not trying to achieve your own happiness, and stress from doing things out of obligation instead of love.

This position can be very relaxing and comforting and reduces tension in the shoulders.

POSITION 5 *(Fifth Chakra—Throat)*

Extend your hands in a cup position, fingers slightly touching, hovering in front of the receiver's neck. **Note:** Do not touch the throat area. Keep your hands about one to two inches away.

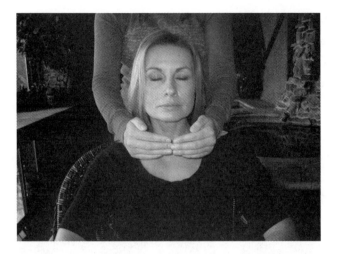

Work here may be helpful for difficulties such as feeling restricted or under pressure, repressed guilt, inability to express oneself, anger or frustration in a situation, being controlling or judgmental, inability to follow through on your needs, addiction, or lack of authority.

POSITION 6 *(Fourth Chakra—Heart)*

Stand behind the receiver and gently place your hands on the left and right sides of the upper chest above the heart.

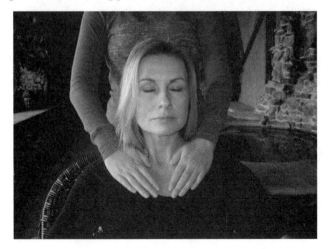

Difficulties in this area are associated with feeling defenseless, problems accepting new ideas, self-criticism and self-centeredness, the inability to have self-love, hatred, depression, or feeling suffocated.

POSITION 7 *(Fourth Chakra—Heart)*

Stand to the **right or left** of the receiver. Gently place your **right** or left hand over the center of the chest (not touching the receiver) and place your **left** or right hand on the upper back, above the shoulder blades.

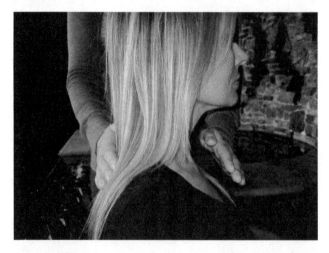

Problems in this area may reflect difficulty giving love, an inability to forgive or trust, and fear of loneliness, denying one's own needs, or taking things too seriously.

POSITION 8 *(Fourth Chakra—Heart)*

Keep your **right** or left hand at the center of the receiver's chest (heart center), lift and move the **left** or right hand down the back to between the shoulder blades directly opposite your other hand.

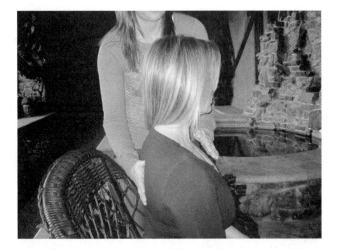

Work here may be helpful for such difficulties as emotional insecurity, grief, jealousy, lack of compassion, loss of hope, doing too much to make others happy, fear of change, or fear of commitment.

POSITION 9 *(Fourth Chakra—Heart)*

Gently place both of your hands at the receiver's chest above the breast area but not touching, your **left** hand on the receiver's right side and your **right** hand on their left side.

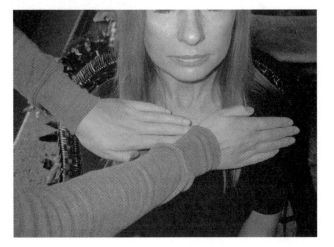

Difficulties in this area may be associated with seeking love by doing for others, betrayal, disappointment, lack of passion for life, fear of suffering or death, repressed anger, jealousy, or envy.

POSITION 10

Gently lift your hands and move them down to the breast area, positioning one of your hands over each breast, but keeping each hand hovering one to two inches away from the body.

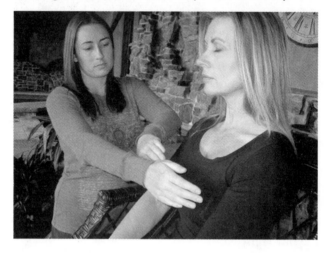

Problems in this area may be associated with such difficulties as mother or father issues: unresolved issues with your own mother or father, mothering others too much, difficulty in letting go, a feeling of resentment or obligation when helping others, or asking too much of yourself.

POSITION 11 *(Third Chakra—Solar Plexus)*

Lift your **right** hand and place it on the receiver's solar plexus area (below the breast) and move your **left** hand into the middle of the receiver's back directly opposite your right hand.

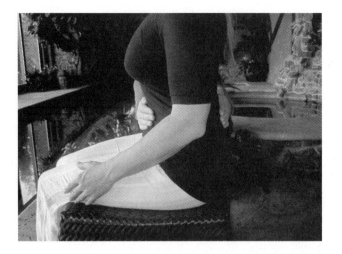

Problems in this area may be associated with weakness of character, lack of self-confidence, inability to handle a crisis, trying to control others, overly high expectations and ambition, repressed anger, lack of self-respect, rigidity, sensitivity to criticism, fear of rejection, feeling powerless, worrying about others, lack of courage, inner conflict, or dependence on approval.

POSITION 12 *(Third Chakra—Solar Plexus; Second Chakra—Sacral)*

Gently place your hands side by side with thumbs touching over the middle and lower abdomen areas.

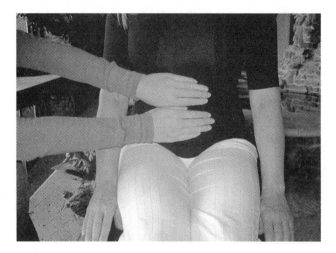

Difficulties in this area may be associated with indecisiveness, intimidation, inability to let oneself be loved, control issues, fear of lack of money, problems with letting go of past issues, or sexual problems.

POSITION 13 *(First Chakra—Root)*

Keeping your hands side by side, lift them and position them hovering approximately two inches above the pubic and genitalia area.

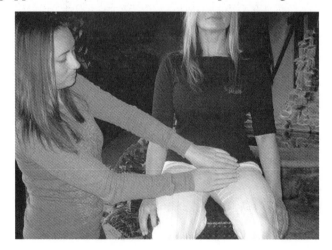

Problems in this area may be associated with unresolved issues with the family, superstitions, lack of loyalty, fear of loss of freedom, difficulties letting go of old belief systems, or resentment.

NOTE: POSITIONS 14, 15, 20, 21, and 24 may help *boost the receiver's immune system.*

"Running the energy" throughout the long bones of the arms and legs sends positive and strengthening energy flowing throughout the entire body. The entire body feels connected and energized.

POSITION 14

Gently take the receiver's right hand in your **right** hand, palm to palm, thumbs interlocking, and place your **left** hand on top of the elbow. This will run the energy from the **HAND** to the **ELBOW**.

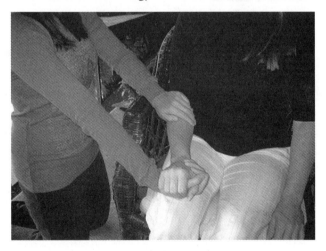

This region may be associated with such problems as difficulty in expressing your needs, self-criticism, a lack of flexibility, resentment, or anger.

POSITION 15

Remove your **left** hand from the elbow and place it on the receiver's shoulder while continuing to hold the right hand in your own. This runs the energy from **HAND** to **SHOULDER**.

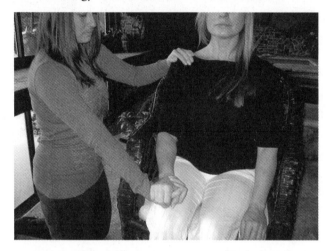

Difficulties in this area may be the result of problems with embracing others, giving and receiving, doubting your capabilities, or being emotionally burdened.

POSITION 16

Place the receiver's hands on the lap. Place both of your hands, side by side, thumbs touching, on the right thigh.

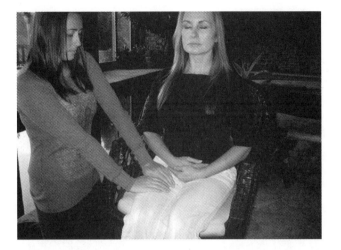

Problems in this area may be associated with difficulty going with the flow of life or fear of moving forward.

POSITION 17

Cup the receiver's knee with both hands, placing your **left** hand under the knee and your **right** hand on top of the knee. Hold firmly but gently.

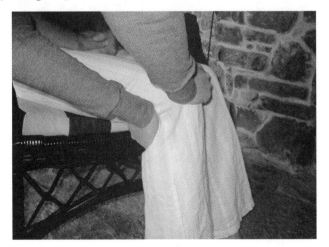

This area may be associated with such problems as inflexibility, stubbornness, or not wanting to move forward in life.

POSITION 18

Gently continue down to the lower leg area, placing your **left** hand behind the leg and your **right** hand in front of the leg midway between the knee and ankle. Lift each of your hands when shifting to this new position.

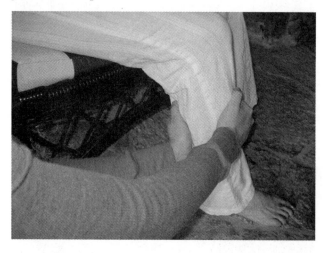

Difficulties in this area may be associated with immobility and issues with "going forward."

POSITION 19

Lift your hands to the next position at the right ankle, keeping your **left** hand behind the ankle and your **right** hand in front and on top of the ankle.

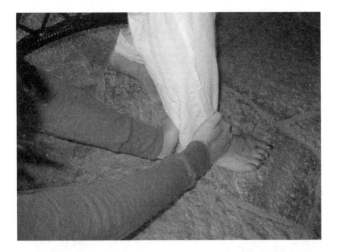

Problems in this area may be due to feeling immobile, not knowing in which direction to proceed, or feeling impeded.

POSITION 20

Run the energy from the **ANKLE** to the **KNEE**, moving your **left** hand to the knee and keeping your **right** hand in front and on top of the ankle.

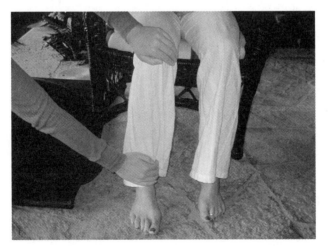

Trouble here may be associated with feeling held back or frustration with someone.

POSITION 21

Run the energy from the **ANKLE** to the **HIP** area. Move your **left** hand to the receiver's hip while keeping your **right** hand in front and on top of the ankle.

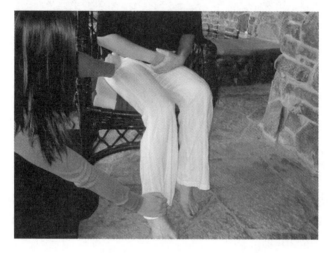

Difficulties in this area may be related to an inability to get away from an unpleasant situation or relationship or the inability to allow life to flow.

> **VERY IMPORTANT NOTE:** *You are now finished on either the right or left side (on whichever side you began) of the receiver. Stand up and walk behind the chair to start on their opposite side. Do not walk in front of this person. You may have released blocked energy that is now flowing outward and to the front from the body through this person's feet and hands. You do not want to bring this energy into your body. Set the intention to send the energy in front of the receiver down to Mother Earth with love and light and healing.*

Now proceed on that opposite side. START FROM POSITION 14 and REPEAT POSITIONS 14 THROUGH 21. When you are finished, proceed to POSITION 22.

POSITION 22

Stand behind the receiver. Gently tilt the receiver forward and place your **left** hand on the left shoulder blade and your **right** hand on the right shoulder blade.

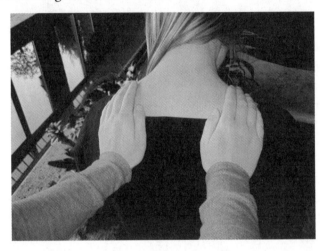

Problems in this area may be associated with the feeling of carrying a burden, of not enough support, or hesitancy in giving affection.

POSITION 23

Lift both hands and gently place them on the lower back of the receiver just above the waist over the adrenal area.

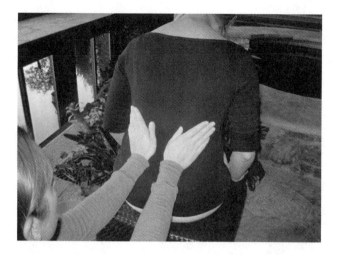

Trouble here may be associated with a constant state of worry, lack of self-worth, or internal chaos.

POSITION 24

With the receiver bent a little forward, place your **right** hand at the base of the neck and your **left** hand at the end of the spine near the tailbone area.

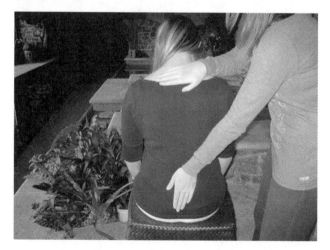

This position runs the energy **UP THE SPINE** to the **BASE OF THE NECK**. It is preferable if you can place your left hand with the fingers pointing toward the neck (not illustrated). If you unable to do that, place your left hand however is comfortable, since it is the intention to direct the energy upward that is important.

Difficulties in this area relate to support issues or lack thereof or feeling overburdened and being unwilling to admit it.

See chapter 10 for complete instructions on balancing, grounding, closing the aura, and disconnecting using Positions 25 and 26.

POSITION 25

Have the receiver sit back in the chair. First, make sure you sent all unwanted energies down to Mother Earth with love, light, and healing. Then step in front of the receiver, lower yourself down however is comfortable for you, and gently place your **left** hand on the receiver's right foot and your **right** hand on the receiver's left foot. This position is for balancing the chakras and grounding the receiver.

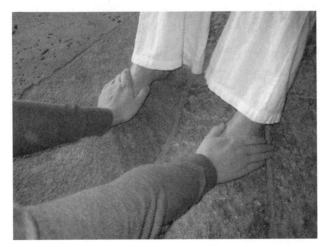

POSITION 26

Again, make sure your intention is to first fill in all the voids that may have been generated during the session with God's healing light. Step behind the receiver. Open both your hands, extend your arms out fully, and place your hands side by side with thumbs touching over the receiver's seventh chakra at the crown of the head. Close and seal the aura.

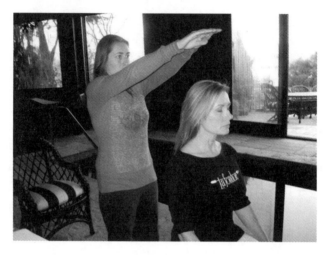

Your treatment is complete. Disconnect from the energy and, if the receiver is sleeping, gently wake them. Ask how they are feeling. Discuss any feelings, sensations, symptoms experienced during the session. Make sure you get the receiver a drink of water after the session. In the next chapter, we'll look at how to close the healing session.

"No person was ever honored for what he received. Honor has been the reward for what he gave."

—CALVIN COOLIDGE

CHAPTER 10

Closing a Session

Because you have opened up so many channels and invited in healing energy, it's important to end a session by closing these channels so that neither you nor your partner picks up any unwanted energies. Before doing any of the next steps, make sure you set your intention and fill in all the voids with God's healing light after your session is complete. You may not be aware of where all of the energy has been released, so simply move around the table or chair and, sweeping your hands in a downward motion, begin at the top of the receiver's head all the way down to the soles of their feet and visualize filling in the voids. Then the next step I recommend is chakra balancing.

1. Balance the Chakras

If you are working with someone sitting in a chair, then you will place your hands on top of their feet. If it has been a table session, your hands go on the soles of the feet. With your intention set to balance the chakras, begin visualizing each chakra on the receiver's body and its corresponding color: red for the root chakra, orange for the sacral chakra, yellow for the solar plexus chakra, green for the heart chakra, blue for the throat chakra, indigo for the third eye chakra, and violet for the crown chakra, in that order. Then ask for each to receive whatever balancing is needed. You can balance your own chakras in this way as well.

2. Ground

Once the chakra balancing is complete, you must ground the receiver. By this I mean center them once again in Mother Earth. If you forget this step, it will cause a feeling of light-headedness, floating, or just being out of sorts.

When you are doing a **self-healing treatment**, after you have balanced your chakras keep your hands on top of your feet. Ask to be grounded to Mother Earth for calm, balance, and whatever your body and spirit may need.

When doing a **table session,** after you have balanced the chakras, keep both your hands on the soles of the receiver's feet and ask God to ground them to Mother Earth and to keep this person centered, balanced, and grounded along with whatever else their body and spirit may need.

When doing a **chair session,** the receiver's feet will be flat on the floor. Keep your hands on the top of both feet and ask God to ground this person to Mother Earth and to keep them centered, balanced, and grounded along with whatever else their body and spirit may need.

Grounding operates like a tree with its roots dug deep into the earth, keeping it balanced and connected so that storms cannot topple it. This technique gathers together all of your energies—physical, emotional, mental, and spiritual. It calms your thoughts and brings about inner harmony and balance. It also helps you to accomplish not only your daily goals but also your spiritual ones too.

I think of grounding as essential to everyday life. Regardless of your religious beliefs, this simple technique can make a huge difference in your life. Whenever you feel spacey or disoriented, it is a good idea to ground yourself, because it keeps you connected to the earth energies.

Grounding relaxes us mentally and emotionally. In an ungrounded state, we might experience nervousness, restlessness, stress, emotional irritability, frenzied euphoria, anxiety, and insomnia.

Grounding also relaxes us physically. In an ungrounded state, we might experience headaches, temperature extremes (e.g., cold or hot skin), muscle spasms and trembling, excessive perspiration, difficulties in breathing or digestion, stinging sensations, and abnormal heart rhythms.

Grounding means we are alert. In an ungrounded state, we might experience dreaminess and a continual semi-trance condition. When we are grounded, we can concentrate mentally. In an ungrounded state, we might experience spaciness and an inability to focus our attention.

When we are grounded, we feel a warm association with our physical body. In an ungrounded state, we might experience cold skin, awkward movements, and strange unfamiliarity with our body, a sensation that we are floating *outside* our body, and the disassociation which is characteristic of the schizoid or schizophrenic condition.

When we are grounded, we feel a secure connection to the physical world. In an ungrounded state, we might experience sensory distortions; for example, muffled hearing, a numb sense of touch, and a dreamlike sense of vision.

When we are grounded, we sense a comfortable connection to other people. In an ungrounded state, we might experience paranoia, hypersensitivity to the presence of other people, an "energy drain" when we are in public, a generally dysfunctional personality, and a belief that we are profoundly different from other people—or even that we are inhuman.

Grounding can be as simple as visualizing your feet with roots growing from the soles all the way down into Mother Earth. Or you can try the following visualization.

GROUNDING VISUALIZATION—
USEFUL ANYTIME YOU FEEL IRRITABLE OR SPACEY

Sit comfortably in a straight-backed chair with your feet flat on the floor and your hands separated and resting on your lap. Keep your hands and feet apart to allow your energy to flow freely.

Sit with your spine as straight as you can.

Now focus your attention on your breath, gently inhaling and exhaling for the next several seconds.

As you allow your eyes to close, feel your body beginning to relax as you continue to breathe.

Visualize roots coming from the soles of your feet.

Feel the roots growing and reaching all the way down into Mother Earth.

Feel the roots taking hold deep in the earth and connecting you securely to the center of the planet.

For a moment, allow your feet-roots to absorb water and nutrients and feel these energies moving up into your legs and body.

As you feel your legs firmly anchored to the ground and the energies branching upward and outward, visualize those energies moving safely into your heart.

Now visualize the energy from heaven (the Divine) coming in through the top of your head and connecting to the earth energies at your heart.

Now feel your entire body being connected with the grounding of Mother Earth and heaven's intuitive energies.

Feel the balance and peace within your inner self.

When you are ready, open your eyes.

It is that simple . . .

3. Close the Aura

The next step is to close the aura. The purpose of this step is to prevent the loss of and to seal in the healing energy just received. This helps to begin the healing process.

When you are doing **self-healing treatments,** ask God to keep your healing energy in and to seal and close your own aura. The intention to do this will allow it to happen.

When you are treating someone on a **table,** stand to the receiver's right, placing your hands as high as you can above the middle of the body. Move your arms over the entire body in a sweeping, circular motion toward the head, then down to the feet, as if you were surrounding this person in a sphere.

Then move back to the middle of the body where you began. Do this three times without stopping, making a large circle around the receiver and visualizing a sphere of white and golden protective light surrounding the entire body.

As you do this, ask God to keep the healing energy in this body, seal the aura of any leaks, and close the aura. When you feel the aura is closed, give thanks for the healing received. Then gently put your hand on the shoulder of the receiver to rouse that person from the relaxed state or even sleep.

When working on someone **seated in a chair,** stand behind the receiver and place your hands above the crown chakra. Keep your hands together and in a sweeping motion make a large circle around the receiver while visualizing a sphere of white and golden light around the entire body.

Ask God to keep the healing energy in this body, seal the aura of any leaks, and close the aura. When you feel the aura is closed, give thanks for the healing received. Then gently put your hand on the shoulder of the receiver to rouse that person from the relaxed state or even sleep.

4. Give Thanks

After completing a session on yourself or someone else, always give thanks to God, your higher self, archangels, angels, spirit guides, and loved ones for the healing received. We want to acknowledge their help because it is God and his helpers that do the healing; we are simply the channel for the energy for ourselves or for the other person. Remember the energy comes from the Divine and passes from our crown chakra down through our heart and into the palms of our hands.

5. Disconnect from the Energy

When doing energy work, it is always important to disconnect from the energy after completing a treatment, whether it is on **yourself or another person**. One way to disconnect the energy is to wipe both hands across each other a few times and ask that the energy be disconnected from yourself or the receiver.

Another way to disconnect is to bring both hands together, fingertips touching, palms apart forming a triangle. Blow between the thumb and index finger (away from the receiver) directed toward the floor or out of a window. Ask to disconnect from the energy. It is also advisable to wash your hands with cold water after a session. This also disconnects the energy.

6. Discuss the Session with the Receiver and Provide Water

You have now completed your entire treatment. It is at this point you wake the receiver (if asleep) by gently placing your hand on a shoulder and softly saying that person's name and "we are all done with your session." Allow the receiver to sit up at the edge of the table for a few minutes to collect thoughts and impressions. Offer the person a glass of cold water. The water is a nice gesture and people tend to be thirsty after the treatment. Always advise people to drink a lot of water for a few days after a session so that any toxins will be released from the body. Ask the receiver how they feel and what physical symptoms or mental, emotional, or spiritual sensations were experienced during the session.

Many times, an issue totally different from the initial reason for the treatment may present itself. This should be discussed to allow the receiver to express any issues of concern. This will help address issues that may have been blocking the flow of energy and causing symptoms and/or disease. If the receiver does not want to discuss the treatment, respect their wishes but offer assistance if they should need you in the future.

Remember: The intention is what brings the energy in, protects, grounds, seals, closes the aura, and disconnects the energy.

The session is now complete.

> *"To become different from what we are, we must have some awareness of what we are."*
> —ERIC HOFFER

CHAPTER 11

Final Thoughts

As you enter into the world of energy healing, see within yourself that stable center, that perfect seed, the perfection, your potential. Allow yourself to move inward to the center and the core of your being. At the core of your very being, there is a diamond of perfection. The universal light, the light of love, is within you.

As this light reflects from the diamond of perfection, you see your potential, your endless abilities, and your expanding talents. Allow yourself to clearly perceive the value in what you have to contribute. Give yourself full permission to do healing work. There is no need for you to wait until you are "perfect" to begin to heal others.

Every one of us needs to heal on all levels. Whether you are well or not, you can do healing work on another as long as you truly believe. It is important to have many kinds of healers at different levels of understanding. Those who have similar understanding and feelings, with whom you resonate, will be drawn to you, and you will be able to learn much from one another.

The most essential ingredients in healing others are your intention to help and the person's desire and permission for you to help. Remember that we are all healers: we not only allow love to come through us, we are love. We do not heal another: the primary source of healing is always within each of us.

Healing is often an up-and-down process. Two steps forward, one step back gives our consciousness time to clearly observe our life. This produces a strong interlocking stitch that will never tear apart again. Experience of an instantaneous healing—creating a life with no seams, no ups and downs—remains in the eternal moment, where all is possible. Treating ourselves and others is a reminder of our natural state and the importance of bringing this healing energy of love into our daily lives.

The first step is to realize that it is a wonderful gift you have given yourself. By reading this book and practicing the Gentle Energy Touch method, you are now ready to begin a journey of self-healing and the healing of others. You are now a channel for the energy of the universal spirit, the Divine. The Divine energy that seemed so mysterious and obscure is, as we now know, quite simple and readily available to us just for the asking. It is with us all the time.

We appear to be standing on the edge of mass spiritual awareness and the desire for growth. Our values, our sense of purpose in life, and the path we should take can no longer be denied by the negative factors that weaken our wellness. Healing our negative behavior and creating a positive attitude allow us to become balanced and healthy. Wellness is the right and privilege of everyone. There is no precondition other than your own free choice to do so.

It's time to **take responsibility** for the **choices you've created.** It's time for self-awareness, newly formed decisions, and a true commitment. Make a commitment to *forgive, to be nonjudgmental, and to love yourself for who you are.*

Healing will allow you to understand your strengths and weaknesses. What has happened to you in the past does not equal your future unless you allow it to. You have the choice—to be sad, angry, violent, sick, addicted, depressed, etc., or happy and healthy.

Remember, *only **you create** what you want **your life** to be.* You are what you believe. There are no limitations but those you set for yourself. Do not allow personal fears to get in the way of your goals. Set yourself free . . . *free to be who you truly are.*

This first step in learning energy healing is to realize that it is a wonderful gift you have given yourself. ***Empower yourself.*** Recover, renew, and rejuvenate. Begin to transform your own destiny for healing your body, mind, and, ultimately, your spirit.

You are a beautiful human being, you are unique and your loving is a miracle.

Use this special gift you have chosen to develop. Then share it with others; for when we give of ourselves to help others heal, that is truly when we heal ourselves.

Life is an incredible journey. Enjoy it and make every moment count.

To Your New Beginning . . .
Awakening through Self-Healing

WITH LOVE AND LIGHT, Barbara

APPENDIX 1

Affirmations for Enhancing Your Healing Work

Affirmations are a powerful ingredient in positive thinking. They work by embedding positive thoughts into our subconscious mind, and over time they train our minds to think in ways that empower us instead of limiting us. Affirmations are not statements that *you wish to be true;* they are statements that *you must believe are true.*

Affirmations are made because you want to achieve something such as overcoming fear, building your confidence, developing an abundance mind-set, drawing happiness, health, and peace into your life, and much more. The whole point of affirmations is to shift your thoughts and emotions to a more positive place. Affirmations allow you to reach inside your inner self and do some exploring to learn things you may not have realized existed inside yourself.

Your subconscious mind is like the registry of your computer that stores configuration settings and options. Remember your body and mind are connected. When you say negative things to yourself, the subconscious mind does not know what is real or not real, so it sends the messages of negativity to your body and the body reacts in that way. When you say positive words, it thinks those are real too and acts upon those words. Once you realize that you can delete and adjust your way of thinking, your subconscious mind will constantly clear out any negative traces that remain and in its place reprogram your mind with positive thoughts.

Before You Begin

Decide what area of your life you want to work on and then decide what it is exactly that you want.

Always use the present or past tense. Do not use the future tense. You want your mind to know the thing you desire has already happened.

Be positive. Use the most positive terms you can. Never use negatives in affirmations.

Write it down. As you begin creating and using affirmations, write them down so you will remember exactly what you want to say. Keep them short and very specific. Personalize them with your name.

Believe. Always believe that what you are saying is happening. The more you believe, the stronger the affirmation.

Repeat. Repetition helps to set the positive affirmation in your head and in your unconscious being.

Schedule time. Always have a specific time daily set aside for your meditations, affirmations, and visualizations. This will set a pattern for you so you will remember them every day.

Sample Affirmations

Take a look at the sample affirmations below and feel free to use them if they resonate with you. If not, try altering them until they trigger the mind-set and emotional state you are trying to attain. Remember: you have the ability to be able to do anything you set your mind to! Just keep it positive and uplifting.

REMEMBER: As the mind perceives, the body works to create.

AFFIRMATIONS FOR RELEASING ROOT CAUSES

I am releasing destructive thoughts and feelings from my body.

I have made the choice to let go of destructive thoughts from my mind.

I have made the choice to let go of things that no longer serve me.

I have made the choice to release any anger and resentment.

I have made the choice to release fear and worry.

I have made the choice to release anything that does not serve my body, mind, and spirit.

AFFIRMATIONS FOR A HEALTHY WEIGHT AND BODY IMAGE

Today I love my body fully, deeply, and joyfully.

My body has its own wisdom, and I trust that wisdom completely.

I am healthy in all aspects of my being.

I release any negative self-images.

I now make healthy choices.

I have the desire to walk and exercise and help my body be strong.

Today I choose to honor my beauty, my strength, and my uniqueness.

I love the way I feel when I take good care of myself.

AFFIRMATIONS FOR SELF-CONFIDENCE AND SELF-BELIEF

Fear is only a feeling; it cannot hold me back.

I can master anything if I do it enough times.

I believe I have the strength to make my dreams come true.

With a solid plan and a belief in myself, there's nothing I cannot do.

I allow myself to raise my vibration to match my desires and passion.

I allow myself to shine and create what has always been waiting for me.

AFFIRMATIONS FOR ABUNDANCE AND PROSPERITY

I open to the flow of great abundance in all areas of my life.

I always have everything I need.

My grateful heart is a magnet that attracts more of everything I desire.

Prosperity surrounds me, prosperity fills me, and prosperity flows to me and through me.

I have the ability to create the abundance for which my life continuously grows.

My day is filled with limitless potential in joy, abundance, and love.

AFFIRMATIONS FOR LIFE PURPOSE

Today I follow my heart and discover my destiny.

My purpose is to develop and share the best parts of myself with others.

I fulfill my life purpose by starting here, right now.

My life purpose can be whatever I decide to make it.

I trust the wisdom of my inner being.

AFFIRMATIONS FOR INNER PEACE

Peace begins with a conscious choice.

Today I embrace simplicity, peace, and solace.

A peaceful heart makes for a peaceful life.

Peace comes when I let go of trying to control every tiny detail.

I allow myself to breathe and relax and feel the peace within.

AFFIRMATIONS FOR OPPORTUNITY

Today I open my mind to the endless opportunities surrounding me.

Opportunities are everywhere, if I choose to see them.

My intuition leads me to the most lucrative opportunities.

Let each of my experiences today be a gateway to something even better.

There are no limitations to my own inner wisdom and my own special uniqueness.

I have incredibly beautiful treasures within me, and I appreciate my brilliance.

AFFIRMATIONS FOR LOVE

I am ready for a healthy, loving relationship.

I am grateful for the people in my life.

I deserve a loving, healthy relationship.

I deserve to be loved, and I allow myself to be loved.

AFFIRMATIONS FOR HEALING

I am strong and healthy.

My energy and vitality are increasing every day.

Abundant health and wellness are my birthright.

I feel the healing taking place right now at this moment and at this time.

I feel the healing light going through my body, cleansing, repairing, and healing all the damaged areas.

Today nurturing myself is my highest priority.

I sleep soundly at bedtime and wake up in the morning feeling renewed, refreshed, and full of energy for my day.

AFFIRMATIONS FOR INNER CLARITY

My inner voice guides me in every moment.

I am centered, calm, and clear.

Harmony is always a sign that I am balanced from within.

I trust my feelings and insights.

I am courageous, smart, and attractive.

I think only positive, healthy thoughts because I know my body will respond by being healthy and in balance.

AFFIRMATIONS FOR SELF-LOVE

I am free to be me and so I shall be.

I am filled with light, love, and peace.

I treat myself with kindness and respect.

I give myself permission to shine.

I'm proud of all I have accomplished.

Today I give myself permission to be greater than my fears.

I love myself no matter what.

I am lovable just as I am.

Always remember that your thoughts can change your life. Positive affirmations have the power to bring about the circumstances in your life that will allow you to become the person you always desired to be.

> *"The easiest thing in the world to be is you.*
> *The most difficult thing to be is what other people want you*
> *to be. Don't let them put you in that position."*
>
> —Leo Buscaglia

APPENDIX 2

Doing Energy Healing on Others

When you start doing healing work on other people, there are a few important things to bear in mind:

1. The Gentle Energy Touch healer is only responsible for channeling the energy. The receivers are responsible for accepting that energy (consciously and subconsciously) and allowing the healing to take place with beneficial effects.

2. The Gentle Energy Touch healer must always get permission from the person to be healed prior to treatment. Before channeling healing energies, always ask if it is okay to transmit the energy to the receiver. Ideally, a verbal confirmation is best.

   For infants, comatose individuals, and those not able to communicate for other reasons, it is not necessary to get a verbal confirmation because they are unable to give it, but you can ask permission from the person's higher self or being and receive permission prior to giving Gentle Energy Touch. Only give Gentle Energy Touch to someone who agrees to receive it. We must respect the wishes of people to have control over their own bodies whether we feel they need energy healing or not. In an emergency situation, when a patient's desire cannot be communicated and time is of the essence, you may proceed to help them.

3. When treating someone for the first time, it is helpful to be aware of any disorders or surgeries that person has experienced. I always ask, "How may I help you, and is there anything you would like me to know before we begin our session?" Then I listen and stay open (without judgment) to that person's challenges. Taking this step will help you gain more clarity on what needs to heal and where to heal.

4. Prior to your session with another person, you should mention that this person may experience different sensations in the body, such as tingling, throbbing, a change of temperature from heat to cold, feelings of energy leaving the body, uneasiness in certain areas, or nothing at all, but the healing is working. The receiver should try to have no expectations but just be open to the healing.

5. At the beginning of a session, as the receiver is either sitting on a chair or lying on a table, have this person close their eyes and breathe and relax for a few moments. Ask that the receiver visualize that with every breath in, the body is filling with healing light and with every breath out, the body is letting go of any worries, emotions, stress, or whatever is not needed. Then ask the receiver to breathe at a normal rate and just relax and enjoy the session.

   Begin your session in silence. When giving or receiving energy healing, we enter a deeper state of consciousness and are open to receive insight, images, and memories (even of past lives). Talking may be distracting and may cause the receiver to miss the messages that would come through at this deeper level of consciousness.

6. After their session, allow the receiver to rest for a few minutes, then offer a glass of water to help the body release

any toxins. The water helps to raise the energy again if the receiver feels somewhat tired from the session.

7. Then ask how the receiver feels and if this person wants you to talk about what you felt during the session, if anything. However, always remember that although pointing out what you have felt is valuable, you should not diagnose or prescribe unless you are a doctor.

APPENDIX 3

Distant Healing

Sometimes distance prevents someone from coming to us for a healing. In such cases, consider distant healing. It is possible to transmit healing energies over any distance, and this form of healing can be very effective. Have you ever sent out a thought or prayer to someone in need of healing? I am sure you have on many occasions. That is a simple form of distance healing.

The following is an outline by which you can send healing to your friends, family, or even strangers, over a distance. Do not underestimate this simple technique. I have experienced phenomenal results using this, and I know many other people who have also.

Set a date and time when you will contact the person either via phone or Skype. Whether doing healing work by phone or Skype, the healer should visualize the receiver's body and "place" your hands over each area as if they were in front of you.

> Have the receiver choose a quiet place to use as a healing sanctuary and mention it is important not to be interrupted while you are doing a healing.

> Make sure that you will not be interrupted in any way on your end too.

> You should prepare and dedicate a space for distance healing.

> Ground yourself, light candles, and dedicate the healing work for this person.

Have the receiver lie or sit down and have the person set the intentions for the healing the way you would do for an in-person healing.

Call in energy for the receiver as if this person were right in front of you and simply use your power of concentration to feel this person's energy.

Be still and go within and proceed to do the healing. Keep your hands over each area until you feel a change in the flow of energy.

When completed, follow the finishing guidelines for balancing, grounding, and closing the aura as discussed in chapter 10.

When you are finished, give thanks for the healing and contact the receiver so the person is aware that you have completed the session; perhaps you may want to talk about what you found and/or what was experienced from the session.

There are many other ways to use distant healing:

1. When I see an ambulance with flashing lights and it could mean the difference between life and death, I ask for healing energies for whomever is in the ambulance, and I quickly visualize God's white and healing light surrounding the ambulance and those inside.

2. I do the same for victims of natural disasters. It can help those who are suffering and also those who have died, as it will ease their passage on to the other realms.

3. For rescue workers at natural disasters, I ask for healing energy to give them greater strength and inspiration to continue with their courageous work of rescuing others.

4. You can send healing energies to Mother Earth. I visualize the earth in both my hands, and I send healing energies to her. I ask for peace, understanding, and whatever comes to

my mind, and I develop a healing consciousness to all that is around me.

5. When I see an animal that has been killed on the street or anywhere, I always ask God to reach for its soul and embrace it in his arms, and I send love, light, and healing to it so that it goes to the light in peace and heals from the trauma.

Remember, it is the intention that sends forth healing energies, and this can be done anywhere and to anyone and anything.

> *"We see the brightness of a new page where*
> *everything yet can happen."*
> —RAINER MARIA RILKE

APPENDIX 4

How to Charge for Your Work

If you decide to continue this work as a professional, you will want to consider the value you place on your work. I strongly recommend an equal exchange for services rendered. We tend to devalue goods and services when we do not pay for them. Receiving money for healing work is payment for your time and the attention you give the client. We may also exchange energy in the form of bartered services. Being able to receive payment for a treatment, without feeling awkward, is a lesson to be learned by the healer. Always respect yourself.

Keep Documentation

When you begin to do Gentle Energy Touch sessions with clients, it is advisable to keep documentation from each session. This confidential information should be maintained on every client. Indicate your findings, what type of treatment was done, and any follow-up. The purpose of the documentation is to assist in recalling what transpired at the last session and help you to compare the assessment with that of the next session. This will allow you and the client to evaluate and understand the progress that is taking place. You can then engage in a more meaningful form of communication with the client. Your client's confidentiality must be respected at all times.

You may not need all the information on the client forms provided in appendix 5, but it will be a good way to document what you do each session. Make copies and utilize them. Keep both forms together in a filing cabinet.

APPENDIX 5

Suggested Client Information Form

I use a form for each new client, and it looks something like this:

Welcome to your Gentle Energy Touch session. Remember, the body has the ability to heal itself, and that healing can be greatly enhanced by relaxing your body as much as possible. Long-term imbalances in the body sometimes require multiple sessions to allow the body to replenish its life force energy and to bring the system back into balance. Self-improvement requires a commitment and a willingness to make positive changes. In order for the Gentle Energy Touch treatment to be effective, you must follow the program and commit to your own self-improvement.

Finally, Gentle Energy Touch practitioners do not diagnose nor do we prescribe medication. A Gentle Energy Touch treatment does not take the place of medical treatment. It is recommended that you see a physician or licensed health care professional for any physical or psychological ailment that you may have.

Please supply the following information:

Date: _____

Print Name: _____

Address: _____

City: _____ State: _____ Zip: _____

Home Phone: _____ Cell: _____

Email: _____

Date of birth: _____

Occupation: _____

Reason for coming: _____

_____

Pertinent medical history (optional): _____

_____

List treatments or medications currently receiving:_____

_____

Medication or Treatment Type: _____

Dosage: _____

When did you start taking? _____

Additional comments: _____

_____

Please Complete: Comments after Gentle Energy Touch Session (optional): _____

_____

_____

APPENDIX 6

Gentle Energy Touch Session Documentation Form

CONFIDENTIAL

Client Name: _____

Session #: _____ Date: _____

Treatment Start time: _____ End time: _____

Treatment Type: *(indicate treatment time for all that apply)*

Scanning & Sweeping _____

Energy Healing _____

Chakra Balancing _____

Aura Clearing _____

Meditation/Visualization _____

Advanced Energy Clearing _____

PRACTITIONER'S TREATMENT NOTES

Indicate the reason(s) the client has come to you. Specify the areas where blockages and/or releases were felt. Identify blockages in the appropriate energy body: physical, emotional, or mental. Has there been any change in client condition, medications or dosages (recommended by doctor), other treatment programs, or environment, etc., that should be noted?

Practitioner Signature _____

Date _____

FURTHER RESOURCES

Scanning and Sweeping Table Video:
http://motivateyourlife.net/sweeping-on-table-mp4/

Scanning and Sweeping Chair Video:
http://motivateyourlife.net/sweeping-on-chair-mp4/

Free Meditation MP3: Relax, Restore, Rebalance:
http://motivateyourlife.net/free-relax-restore-rebalance-mp3/

Free Meditation MP3: Building Self-Confidence:
http://motivateyourlife.net/free-building-self-confidence-mp3/

Free Meditation MP3: Empower Your Potential:
http://motivateyourlife.net/free-empower-your-potential-passion-mp3/

Helpful Websites

www.DailyOM.com

www.HealingTouchInternational.org

www.Lifetransformationsecrets.com

www.MotivateYourLife.Net

www.OrinDaben.com

Helpful Books

Lise Bourbeau, *Your Body's Telling You: Love Yourself!* (Lotus Press, 2002)

Master Choa Kok Sui, *Practical Psychic Self-Defense for Home and Office* (Institute for Eastern Studies, 2009)

Master Stephen Co and Eric B. Robins, MD, *Your Hands Can Heal You: Pranic Healing Energy Remedies to Boost Vitality and Speed Recovery from Common Health Problems* (Atria Books, 2004)

Louise Hay, *Heal Your Body* (Hay House, 1984)

Louise Hay, *The Power Is Within You* (Hay House, 1991)

Louise Hay, *You Can Heal Your Life* (Hay House, 1984)

Esther and Jerry Hicks, *Ask and It Is Given* (Hay House, 2010)

Carolyn Myss, *Advanced Energy Anatomy* (audio CD) (Sounds True, 2001)

Carolyn Myss, *Anatomy of the Spirit* (Harmony, 1997)

Carolyn Myss, *Energy Anatomy* (audio CD) (Sounds True, 2001)

Carolyn Myss, *Sacred Contracts* (Harmony, 2003)

Carolyn Myss, *Why People Don't Heal and How They Can* (Harmony, 1998)

Doreen Virtue, *Angel Numbers 101* (Hay House, 2008)

Doreen Virtue, *Daily Guidance from Your Angels* (Hay House, 2006)

Doreen Virtue, *Healing with the Angels* (Hay House, 1999)

Music to Listen to When Doing Healing

Ron Allen, *Yoga* (Solitudes, 1999)

Robert Haig Coxon, *Prelude to Infinity* (Music Design, 2005)

Robert Haig Coxon, *The Silent Path* (Music Design, 1996)

Deuter, *Koyasan: Reiki Sound Healing* (New Earth Records, 2007)

Deuter, *Reiki Hands of Light* (New Earth Records, 2002)

Deuter, *Spiritual Healing* (New Earth Records, 2008)

Steven Halpern, *Inner Peace* (Inner Peace Music, 2002)

Steven Halpern, *Music for Healing Mind, Body & Spirit* (Relaxation, 2003)

Michael Maxwell, *Nature's Spa: Soothing Massage* (Solitudes, 2001)

Acknowledgments

There comes a time in your life when you finally become aware of what life is really about and the importance of nonmaterial things. When love is all around you, you realize how wealthy you are. My being healthy and having a loving relationship with God, family, and friends are the most important things in the world. I thank God every day for all that I am.

Thank you, Harold, my dear and loving husband, for always being there for me. To our children, John Savin and Sandra Parracino, thank you for being supportive and for truly listening. The greatest and most precious gift from God is a child. I love you both with all my heart and soul. To my first grandchild, Kyla, I love when you lay your head on my shoulder and fall asleep. The hugs and kisses always brighten my day. Grandma loves you more than words can say. To my second grandchild, Kaden, born September 7, four days after my birthday; I love the way you look into my eyes, then touch my face. I just melt. Grandma loves you more than words can say. I mention four days after my birthday because Grandma Jenny, my mom, and I all were born on September 3 . . . amazing! By the time my book is published, I will be a grandma for the third time . . . I am so excited. It is the first child for my son, John, and his wife, Nelly.

To my father, Frank Babich, now in heaven with my mom—I know both of you are celebrating. Mom waited eight years for you. To my mom, Sally, who passed away on March 2, 2006, thank you for allowing me to do a healing on you the day before you passed on. I love you both with all my heart and miss you very much. To my sister, Janet, and her husband, Louis, thank you for the privilege of marrying you in March 20, 2004, in Florida; that was truly an honor! I love you.

To Linda Mackenzie, I am very grateful for you helping me get back to God. That was one of the greatest gifts I have ever received. To my Reiki teachers, Margaret Case (rest in peace, Margaret), Yiebah, and Lizette Fernandez (rest in peace, Lizette), there are no words to express the precious gift you have shared with me. May your souls be filled with the true meaning of love, light, and healing.

To Louise Mastromarino and Kathryn Rosenthal, my first Gentle Energy Touch students, thank you both for an experience of a lifetime. You are always in my heart and thoughts, and my love for you will always be. To Dr. Leia Stathakos, thank you for the privilege and opportunity to teach you Gentle Energy Touch and work at the Island Women's Center. You are truly a special person.

To Joan Mazzeo-Little, RN, best friend and second sister; friends who listen are rare treasures. Thank you for your valuable input as I was writing this book and for the opportunity to teach you and your husband, Bill, Gentle Energy Touch. To Cheryl Edwards, my friend, thank you for helping me celebrate the joy of finding the confidence to accomplish writing this book.

To all my nieces and nephews, I love you all. And thanks to my niece Stefanie Cuomo for that day in the metaphysical store. If it weren't for that, I might not be writing this dedication now. I love you, Stefanie.

To my dearest friend Joan Lombardi (my angel in heaven), I miss you and your cooking. You will always be my beautiful rose, Joan. To Sammy, my truly loving Gentle Energy Touch spirit dog, thank you for teaching me the true meaning of what unconditional love is about. I will always cherish your funny ways and the love you've brought to me as I was writing this book. Sammy, you will never be forgotten and will be forever in my heart.

To my Grandma Jenny, thank you for doing energy healing on me . . . I truly now understand what you were doing. To my Grandma Rose, thank you for teaching me what giving of yourself unconditionally by volunteering means. This has taught me so much about healing myself and others. I will always be grateful and love and miss you both.

Just a note: it has taken me many years to finish this book. We have been living in California since February 2004. I am truly living my purpose. I currently work for the California Health & Longevity Institute (since January 2007) located in The Four Seasons Hotel in Westlake Village, California. I am the energy healing specialist and clinical and medical hypnotherapist. I also work for the Mind, Body, and Spirit Center with Dr. Sharon Norling, author of *Your Doctor Is Wrong*.

Who says dreams don't come true?

Thank you, God, for being so patient, for my unconditional love for you, for my commitment to constant growth, and for helping me to teach others how to heal.

Wishing you love, light, and wholeness,
Barbara

About the Author

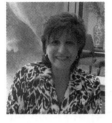

PHOTO BY GERRY FURTH

Barbara E. Savin is an inspirational author and speaker, Gentle Energy Touch specialist, clinical hypnotherapist, certified Reiki master/teacher, and certified Pranic healer.

Since 2007, Barbara has been a consultant at California Health & Longevity Institute, located onsite at Four Seasons Hotel Westlake Village, and now holds the position of Clinical Hypnotherapist and Energy Healing Specialist there. Barbara also provides energy healing sessions as well as clinical and medical hypnosis for individuals, corporations, groups, celebrities, directors, producers, and guests of R4.0 of The Ranch at Live Oak/Malibu and at Dr. Sharon Norling's Mind Body Spirit Center in Westlake Village, CA.

To find out more, please visit her online at *www.BarbaraSavin.com* and on her Facebook page: *facebook.com/GentleEnergyTouch*

To Our Readers

Conari Press, an imprint of Red Wheel/Weiser, publishes books on topics ranging from spirituality, personal growth, and relationships to women's issues, parenting, and social issues. Our mission is to publish quality books that will make a difference in people's lives—how we feel about ourselves and how we relate to one another. We value integrity, compassion, and receptivity, both in the books we publish and in the way we do business.

Our readers are our most important resource, and we appreciate your input, suggestions, and ideas about what you would like to see published.

Visit our website at *www.redwheelweiser.com* to learn about our upcoming books and free downloads, and be sure to go to *www.redwheelweiser.com/newsletter* to sign up for newsletters and exclusive offers.

You can also contact us at *info@rwwbooks.com.*

Conari Press
an imprint of Red Wheel/Weiser, LLC
65 Parker Street, Suite 7
Newburyport, MA 01950
www.redwheelweiser.com

31901059225567